Cannabis Science and Therapeutics

Leah Sera
Carrie Hempel-Sanderoff

Cannabis Science and Therapeutics

The Essential Guide for Clinicians

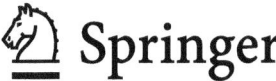 Springer

Leah Sera
Department of Practice, Sciences
and Health Outcomes Research
University of Maryland School of
Pharmacy
Baltimore, MD, USA

Carrie Hempel-Sanderoff
Department of Practice, Sciences
and Health Outcomes Research
University of Maryland School of
Pharmacy
Baltimore, MD, USA

ISBN 978-3-031-80351-2   ISBN 978-3-031-80352-9   (eBook)
https://doi.org/10.1007/978-3-031-80352-9

Editorial Contact: Jessica Chio
This Springer imprint is published by the registered company Springer Nature
Switzerland AG
The registered company address is: Gewerbestrasse 11, 6330 Cham, Switzerland

If disposing of this product, please recycle the paper.

Preface

The first time I really thought about cannabis as medicine was in 2010 as a postgraduate clinical pharmacy resident participating in a rotation at a local hospice organization. During morning rounds (where the healthcare team discusses each patient before going their separate ways for the day), one nurse mentioned that a terminally ill cancer patient asked her about using cannabis to manage symptoms. At that time, Maryland was still a few years away from enacting legislation to permit medical use of cannabis. There was no legal way for this patient to access a potentially beneficial therapeutic modality, and no one on the team (including me) was very knowledgeable about the risks and benefits of using cannabis. As a dedicated pharmacy resident, I started to dig into the available research related to medical cannabis and, over the next several years, would have occasion to educate patients or their caregivers about the topic if they brought it up during a consult while I practiced as a clinical pharmacist on a palliative medicine team at a local hospital.

In 2017, as a faculty member at the University of Maryland School of Pharmacy, I was excited to learn that our dean wanted to create a master's program in medical cannabis science. I asked my department chair to put in a word on my behalf with the dean so that I could perhaps teach a course in this new program. After bringing some of my ideas for what this program might look like, the dean asked me to spearhead the proposal, development, and implementation of the program, a project that has been one of the most challenging and rewarding of my career so far as an educator. Since the program launched in

2019, I have devoted much of my professional life to educating students, healthcare professionals, and policymakers about how cannabis-based medicines might be safely used for the benefit of patients. Cannabis is medicine; as such, there are benefits and risks to consider for individual patients, as well as legal and regulatory matters and public health concerns.

This book is intended as both a quick reference for clinicians and a source of background information on the scientific, clinical, and regulatory aspects of the medical cannabis field. The legal landscape in the United States and worldwide is in flux; with greater access comes greater responsibility (please pardon the superhero allusion; I'm a boy mom). Clinicians should be prepared to ask about cannabis use and discuss it knowledgeably and empathetically. Although medical and non-medical cannabis use are both more widely accepted in today's culture, stigma remains and prevents both clinicians and patients from discussing cannabis use openly. As clinicians, we should do everything we can to reduce this stigma, starting with examining our biases and the depth of our scientific and clinical knowledge. I hope that you find this book a helpful resource that aids you in providing optimal care to your patients.

From one lifelong learner to another. - Leah

Baltimore, MD, USA   Leah Sera
September 2024

Contents

About the Authors

Leah Sera is an Associate Professor in the Department of Practices Sciences and Health Outcomes Research and Associate Dean for Recruitment, Admissions, and Integration at the University of Maryland School of Pharmacy. She was the inaugural program director of the Master of Science in Cannabis Science and Therapeutics (MCST) program, the first of its kind in the country, from 2019 to 2024. Dr. Sera received her PharmD from the University of Maryland School of Pharmacy in 2010. She is a board-certified pharmacotherapy specialist and has served as a clinical pharmacist on palliative medicine and transitional care teams. Dr. Sera has been invited to speak on pain management, palliative medicine, and cannabis therapeutics at professional medical and pharmacy conferences and medical centers such as the National Institutes of Health. Her research interests include health disparities, medical cannabis utilization, pharmaceutical health policy, and the scholarship of teaching and learning. She lives in Olney, MD, with her husband, four sons, three cats, two dogs, and a bearded dragon, and spends her free time watching youth sports, practicing yoga, reading, and gardening.

Carrie Hempel-Sanderoff is a physician who has spent her career caring for critically ill and terminally ill patients. During that time, her attention has been drawn to the space of suffering between the pharmaceuticals, procedures, and technology of medicine. An emerging theme was that patients with chronic and life-threatening illnesses experience holistic pain, symptoms, and suffering that is often unaddressed. Dr. Hempel-Sanderoff's training as an osteopathic physician has led her to embrace and explore the uses of complementary and alternative therapies to improve her patients' comfort and quality of life. In 2018, she opened a symptom management practice to assist and educate patients in the community about medical cannabis. In 2020, she joined the University of Maryland School of Pharmacy's MCST program as an adjunct faculty member and has collaborated with her pharmacist colleagues in course development, clinical practice, and authorship. Dr. Hempel-Sanderoff currently works as a hospice physician in Baltimore, MD, and continues to teach in the MCST program. She lives with her husband Brian, a pharmacist, and a spoiled Great Dane. When she's not at work, you can find her on the sidelines of her son's travel baseball team, trying not to embarrass him with her cheering.

Abbreviations

2-AG	2-Arachidonylglycerol
5-HT	Serotonin
AEA	N-Arachidonoylethanolamide
AIDS	Acquired immunodeficiency syndrome
ASD	Autism spectrum disorder
CB	Cannabinoid
CBC	Cannabichromene
CBD	Cannabidiol
CBG	Cannabigerol
CBN	Cannabinol
CHS	Cannabis hyperemesis syndrome
CNS	Central nervous system
COPD	Congestive obstructive pulmonary disease
CSA	Controlled Substances Act
CUD	Cannabis use disorder
CYP	Cytochrome P450
DEA	Drug Enforcement Agency
DOJ	Department of Justice
DSM-5	Diagnostic and Statistical Manual of Mental Disorders
ECS	Endocannabinoid system
FAAH	Fatty acid amide hydrolase
FDA	Food and Drug Administration
GABA	Gamma-aminobutyric acid
GI	Gastrointestinal
GPCR	G-protein-coupled receptor

HHS	Department of Health and Human Services
HIV	Human immunodeficiency virus
MAGL	Monoacylglycerol lipase
MS	Multiple sclerosis
NASEM	National Academies of Sciences, Engineering, and Medicine
NDA	New drug application
NIH	National Institutes of Health
PPAR	Peroxisome proliferator-activated nuclear receptors
PTSD	Post-traumatic stress disorder
PUFA	Polyunsaturated fatty acid
RCT	Randomized controlled trial
THC	Tetrahydrocannabinol
TRP	Transient receptor potential
US	United States
USP	United States Pharmacopeia

The Endocannabinoid System: The Most Important System You Never Learned in School

1.1 Discovery of the Endocannabinoid System

OK, everyone. Raise your hand if you learned about the *endocannabinoid system* (ECS) during pharmacy school (or medical school, nursing school, or dental school). If you didn't raise your hand, don't worry—most of your colleagues in the health professions also didn't have any formal instruction on this biological system that appears to be involved in many physiological processes in humans and other mammals. Only about 9% of medical schools report including content related to the ECS in their curricula [1].

Despite the lack of formal instruction in health professions' curricula, the ECS has been a subject of intense interest and research over the last several decades. In the 1980s, neuroscience researcher Allyn Howlett and her team identified a G-protein-coupled receptor (GPCR) densely distributed in the mammalian brain and central and peripheral nervous system. Surprisingly, this new receptor—the cannabinoid-1 (CB1) receptor—was more prominent than any other receptor discovered thus far [2]. Not long after this, cannabinoid researcher Raphael Mechoulam and his team in Israel identified the molecule that serves as the ligand for this receptor, N-arachidonoylethanolamide (AEA). This

© The Author(s), under exclusive license to Springer Nature Switzerland AG 2025
L. Sera, C. Hempel-Sanderoff, *Cannabis Science and Therapeutics*,
https://doi.org/10.1007/978-3-031-80352-9_1

molecule is more commonly called *anandamide*, a Sanskrit word that translates to "bliss molecule" [3]. A second cannabinoid receptor (CB2) was soon identified in the peripheral tissues and lymphatic immune tissues, followed by the discovery of a second ligand named 2-arachidonylglycerol (2-AG) [3]. These fatty acid neurotransmitters have been named *endocannabinoids* or "endogenous cannabinoids."

1.2   ECS Anatomy: Receptors and Ligands

The ECS is a diverse, diffuse physiologic regulatory system located in every body tissue and system and includes receptors, their ligands, and the enzymes that synthesize and metabolize them. The two major receptors, CB1 and CB2, appear to play an essential role in the function of the central nervous system (CNS), the circulatory system, the gastrointestinal (GI) tract, the reproductive system, and the bone marrow and immune system. CB1 receptors are located most densely in the central and peripheral nervous system. The highly lipophilic endocannabinoids AEA and 2-AG are produced on demand in the post-synapse during excitatory nerve signal transmission (Fig. 1.1). Once released, they travel to pre-synaptic CB receptors and modulate the release of excitatory neurotransmitters such as glutamate [4]. The effect is short-lived; endocannabinoids are quickly broken down in the post-synapse by two unique metabolic enzymes. AEA is broken down by fatty acid amide hydrolase (FAAH), resulting in byproducts of arachidonate and ethanolamine. 2-AG is broken down by monoacylglycerol lipase (MAGL), with byproducts of arachidonate and glycerol [5]. The effect of this cycle is the depression and regulation of excitatory impulses being transmitted throughout the nervous system tissues. Essentially, the ECS acts as a "braking system" for the nervous system's response to a stressful stimulus.

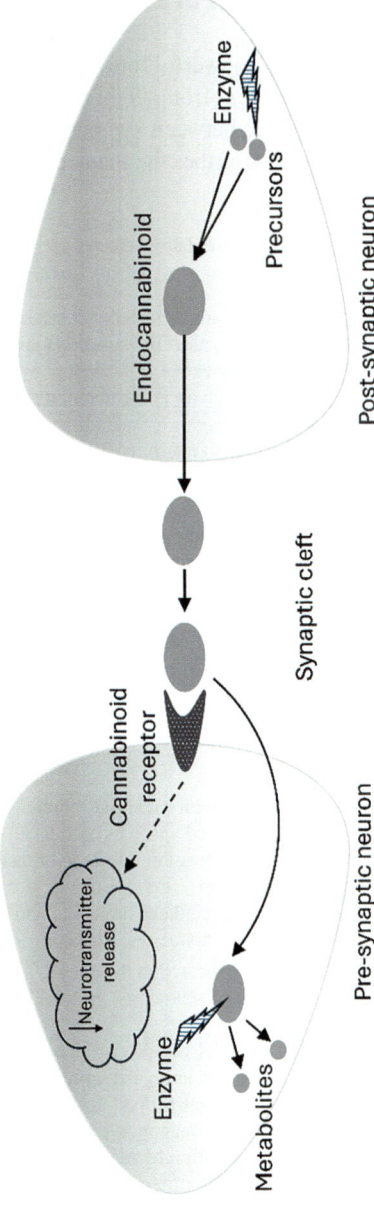

Fig. 1.1 Endocannabinoid synthesis, action, and metabolism

1.3   Physiologic Effects of ECS Activity

Holistically, the ECS plays a powerful role in homeostasis and the transition of the nervous system from "fight or flight" to "rest and digest," restoring the balance between sympathetic and parasympathetic activity. Table 1.1 describes the many physiologic effects of the ECS.

Table 1.1 Physiologic effects of the ECS

Organ system	Effects
CNS [5, 6]	• CB1 receptors are highly concentrated in the brain and spinal cord, and CB2 receptors are present in the CNS to a lesser extent • The primary activity is the maintenance of homeostasis • Protective role in neurogenesis, neuroinflammation, and neurotoxicity • Regulation of neural stem cell growth and division
Cardiovascular [7, 8]	• CB1 receptors in the myocardium influence contractility and cardiac output • CB1 receptors in the endovascular tissue influence smooth muscle proliferation and vasodilation • Activation of CB1 receptors typically reduces blood pressure and increases heart rate • CB2 receptors found in endothelial cells, myocytes, and vascular smooth muscle cells • Anti-inflammatory, antioxidant, and anti-atherogenic effects
Respiratory [9]	• CB1 receptors reduce respiratory rate centrally but do not cause sustained apnea as opioids do • CB1 receptor activation results in bronchial smooth muscle relaxation • CB2 activation regulates bronchial and alveolar immune cells, lymphocytes, and peripheral immune cells
GI tract [10]	• CB1 receptors located in the enteric nervous system influence gastric secretions, gastric emptying, and intestinal motility • Activation of CB1 receptors reduces GI motility and secretions, lowers intragastric pressure, and decreases pyloric muscle contraction • CB1 receptors in vagal nerve pathways decrease gastric acid secretion by reducing histamine release from enterochromaffin cells

(continued)

Table 1.1   (continued)

Organ system	Effects

Reproductive [11, 12]	• CB1 and CB2 receptors present in the hypothalamus, anterior pituitary, and ovaries (HPO axis) and the testis, vas deferens, and spermatozoa
	• AEA and FAAH found in ovaries, endometrium, and myometrium
	• Endogenous and exogenous cannabinoids can:
	  – Disrupt HPO axis signaling
	  – Reduce circulating gonadotropin-releasing hormone (GnRH) levels
	  – Disrupt or prevent ovulation and reduce quality of oogenesis
	  – Decrease sperm motility

Immune [10]	• CB1 and CB2 receptors present in immune cells • Endocannabinoids suppress activation of macrophages • Activation of CB1 and CB2 receptors decreases lymphocyte and inflammatory cytokine synthesis • Endocannabinoids reduce neutrophil aggregation and "cytokine rush," preventing inflammation
Musculoskeletal [13]	• Bone tissue contains high levels of AEA and 2-AG • CB1 receptors in skeletal sympathetic nerve terminals regulate bone formation through adrenergic signaling • CB2 receptors in osteocytes, osteoblasts, and osteoclasts regulate bone turnover, stress, and inflammation • Anandamide increases muscle glucose uptake and insulin signaling • GPR55 and TRPV receptor interactions with the ECS influence osteoclast and osteoblast behavior • CB1 and CB2 activation attenuates inflammatory and neuropathic pain effects

1.4   Say It Three Times, Fast: Endocannabinoidome

As cannabinoid researchers continue exploring the human ECS, an expanded view of the system has emerged, recognizing that endocannabinoid activity involves the modulation of numerous receptors other than CB1 and CB2, including transient receptor potential (TRP) ion channels, peroxisome proliferator-activated nuclear receptors (PPARs), and orphan GPCRs in all organ systems [14]. The National Institutes of Health (NIH) recognized the significance of the ECS in 2006, publishing a review of the widespread physiologic effects of the ECS and therapeutic potential in specific disorders such as mood and anxiety disorders, neurodegenerative and movement disorders, multiple sclerosis, neuropathic pain, seizures, malignancy, and cardiovascular and metabolic disorders [15].

The study of these interactions and their downstream effects has led to the recognition of a more diverse system involving non-CB receptor pathways regulating inflammation, tissue proliferation, and metabolic functioning. This system has been termed the *endocannabinoidome* to more fully capture the true nature and scope of the influence of CB receptors and endocannabinoids.

1.4.1   Nutrients

The endocannabinoidome includes key nutrients that interact with and support the ECS. For instance, polyunsaturated fatty acids (PUFAs) are precursors to AEA and 2-AG and are essential components of cellular anatomy and function. Humans do not synthesize PUFAs; we must supplement these by consuming omega-3 and omega-6 fatty acids [16]. Omega-6 fatty acids are found in corn, cottonseed, and soybean oils and have pro-inflammatory effects, and consumption should be minimized. Omega-3 fatty acids have anti-inflammatory properties and are found in fatty fish such as tuna or salmon or plant sources such as hemp, chia, and flax seeds [17].

1.4.2   Microbiome

Another important component of ECS function is the microbiome. Although unpleasant to think about, the human body is home to a wide variety of bacteria, viruses, and fungal species. In a healthy system, the body and immune system can balance "friendly" colonizers with invasive or "unfriendly" pathogens.

Modern diets, environmental stressors, antibiotics, and medications can all negatively affect the balance of friendly and unfriendly organisms in the gut and body, resulting in inflammation, infection, and metabolic dysfunction. Probiotics increase the concentration of friendly bacteria such as *acidophilus* and *bifidum*, which appear to mimic some endocannabinoid activities. These include anti-inflammatory effects when binding to PPARs and anxiolytic and analgesic effects interacting with CB receptors [18]. Alteration of the gut microbiome by diet or medications (e.g., antibiotics) may up- or downregulate CB receptors or modulate endocannabinoid tone [19]. So far, these studies are just beginning to shine a light on the complex relationship between the ECS, nutrients, and metabolism, and this is likely to be a research topic of great interest in the coming years.

References

1. Evanoff AB, Quan T, Dufault C, Awad M, Bierut LJ. Physicians-in-training are not prepared to prescribe medical marijuana. Drug Alcohol Depend. 2017;180:151–5. https://doi.org/10.1016/j.drugalcdep.2017.08.010.
2. Silver RJ. The endocannabinoid system of animals. Animals. 2019;9(9):686.
3. Rezende B, Alencar AK, de Bem GF, Fontes-Dantas FL, Montes GC. Endocannabinoid system: chemical characteristics and biological activity. Pharmaceuticals. 2023;16(2):148.
4. Zou S, Kumar U. Cannabinoid receptors and the endocannabinoid system: signaling and function in the central nervous system. Int J Mol Sci. 2018;19(3):833. https://doi.org/10.3390/ijms19030833. PMID: 29533978; PMCID: PMC5877694.
5. Wilson RI, Nicoll RA. Endocannabinoid signaling in the brain. Science. 2002;296(5568):678–82. https://doi.org/10.1126/science.1063545.
6. Gao Y, Vasilyev DV, Goncalves MB, Howell FV, Hobbs C, Reisenberg M, Shen R, Zhang MY, Strassle BW, Lu P, Mark L, Piesla MJ, Deng K, Kouranova EV, Ring RH, Whiteside GT, Bates B, Walsh FS, Williams G, Pangalos MN, Samad TA, Doherty P. Loss of retrograde endocannabinoid signaling and reduced adult neurogenesis in diacylglycerol lipase knock-out mice. J Neurosci. 2010;30(6):2017–24. https://doi.org/10.1523/JNEUROSCI.5693-09.2010. PMID: 20147530; PMCID: PMC6634037.

7. Chanda D, Neumann D, Glatz JFC. The endocannabinoid system: overview of an emerging multi-faceted therapeutic target. Prostaglandins Leukot Essent Fatty Acids. 2019;140:51–6. https://doi.org/10.1016/j.plefa.2018.11.016. Epub 2018 Nov 29.
8. Karimian Azari E, Kerrigan A, O'Connor A. Naturally occurring cannabinoids and their role in modulation of cardiovascular health. J Diet Suppl. 2020;17(5):625–50. https://doi.org/10.1080/19390211.2020.1790708. Epub 2020 Jul 17.
9. Wiese BM, Alvarez Reyes A, Vanderah TW, Largent-Milnes TM. The endocannabinoid system and breathing. Front Neurosci. 2023;17:1126004. https://doi.org/10.3389/fnins.2023.1126004. PMID: 37144090; PMCID: PMC10153446.
10. Behl T, Makkar R, Sehgal A, Singh S, Makeen HA, Albratty M, Alhazmi HA, Meraya AM, Bungau S. Exploration of multiverse activities of endocannabinoids in biological systems. Int J Mol Sci. 2022;23(10):5734. https://doi.org/10.3390/ijms23105734. PMID: 35628545; PMCID: PMC9147046.
11. Walker OS, Holloway AC, Raha S. The role of the endocannabinoid system in female reproductive tissues. J Ovarian Res. 2019;12(1):3. https://doi.org/10.1186/s13048-018-0478-9. PMID: 30646937; PMCID: PMC6332911.
12. du Plessis SS, Agarwal A, Syriac A. Marijuana, phytocannabinoids, the endocannabinoid system, and male fertility. J Assist Reprod Genet. 2015;32(11):1575–88. https://doi.org/10.1007/s10815-015-0553-8. Epub 2015 Aug 16. PMID: 26277482; PMCID: PMC4651943.
13. Finn DP, Haroutounian S, Hohmann AG, Krane E, Soliman N, Rice AS. Cannabinoids, the endocannabinoid system, and pain: a review of preclinical studies. Pain. 2021;162(Suppl 1):S5–S25. https://doi.org/10.1097/j.pain.0000000000002268. PMID: 33729211; PMCID: PMC8819673.
14. Daeninck P, Schecter D, Davis MP, Cyr C. Overview of the endocannabinoid system and endocannabinoidome. In: Cannabis and cannabinoid-based medicines in cancer care. Cham: Springer; 2022. p. 1–40.
15. Pacher P, Bátkai S, Kunos G. The endocannabinoid system as an emerging target of pharmacotherapy. Pharmacol Rev. 2006;58(3):389–462. https://doi.org/10.1124/pr.58.3.2. PMID: 16968947; PMCID: PMC2241751.
16. Murff HJ, Edwards TL. Endogenous production of long-chain polyunsaturated fatty acids and metabolic disease risk. Curr Cardiovasc Risk Rep. 2014;8(12):418. https://doi.org/10.1007/s12170-014-0418-1. PMID: 26392837; PMCID: PMC4574498.
17. Komarnytsky S, Rathinasabapathy T, Wagner C, Metzger B, Carlisle C, Panda C, Le Brun-Blashka S, Troup JP, Varadharaj S. Endocannabinoid system and its regulation by polyunsaturated fatty acids and full spectrum

hemp oils. Int J Mol Sci. 2021;22(11):5479. https://doi.org/10.3390/ijms22115479. PMID: 34067450; PMCID: PMC8196941.

18. Rousseaux C, Thuru X, Gelot A, Barnich N, Neut C, Dubuquoy L, Dubuquoy C, Merour E, Geboes K, Chamaillard M, Ouwehand A, Leyer G, Carcano D, Colombel JF, Ardid D, Desreumaux P. Lactobacillus acidophilus modulates intestinal pain and induces opioid and cannabinoid receptors. Nat Med. 2007;13(1):35–7. https://doi.org/10.1038/nm1521. Epub 2006 Dec 10.

19. Srivastava RK, Lutz B, Ruiz de Azua I. The microbiome and gut endocannabinoid system in the regulation of stress responses and metabolism. Front Cell Neurosci. 2022;16:867267. https://doi.org/10.3389/fncel.2022.867267. PMID: 35634468; PMCID: PMC9130962.

The Cannabis Plant: Where It All Begins

2

2.1   What's in a Name?

Before diving into scientific details relating to the botanical science of this plant, we thought it would be helpful to discuss its various names and what they mean. Firstly, the scientific name of this plant is *Cannabis sativa* Linnaeus (so named by legendary taxonomist Carl von Linnaeus). Throughout this text, we will refer to the plant as "cannabis." Specifically, *Cannabis sativa* L. is a botanical species belonging to the family Cannabaceae. The hops plant (used in brewing beer) also belongs to this botanical family [1]. The Linnaean classification of cannabis is illustrated in Fig. 2.1 to provide you with some fun trivia to break out at parties (well, a certain kind of party, perhaps).

"Hemp" is the common English name for *Cannabis sativa* L. This word is derived from the same linguistic root as "cannabis" [2]. Historically, the term "hemp" appears to have described all forms of the plant [3]. However, in modern society, the term "hemp" refers to strains of cannabis that contain less than 0.3% tetrahydrocannabinol (THC), the psychoactive compound in cannabis. This distinction has important legal implications in the United States, where hemp-derived products are not subject to regulation under the Controlled Substances Act (CSA), unlike

© The Author(s), under exclusive license to Springer Nature Switzerland AG 2025
L. Sera, C. Hempel-Sanderoff, *Cannabis Science and Therapeutics*,
https://doi.org/10.1007/978-3-031-80352-9_2

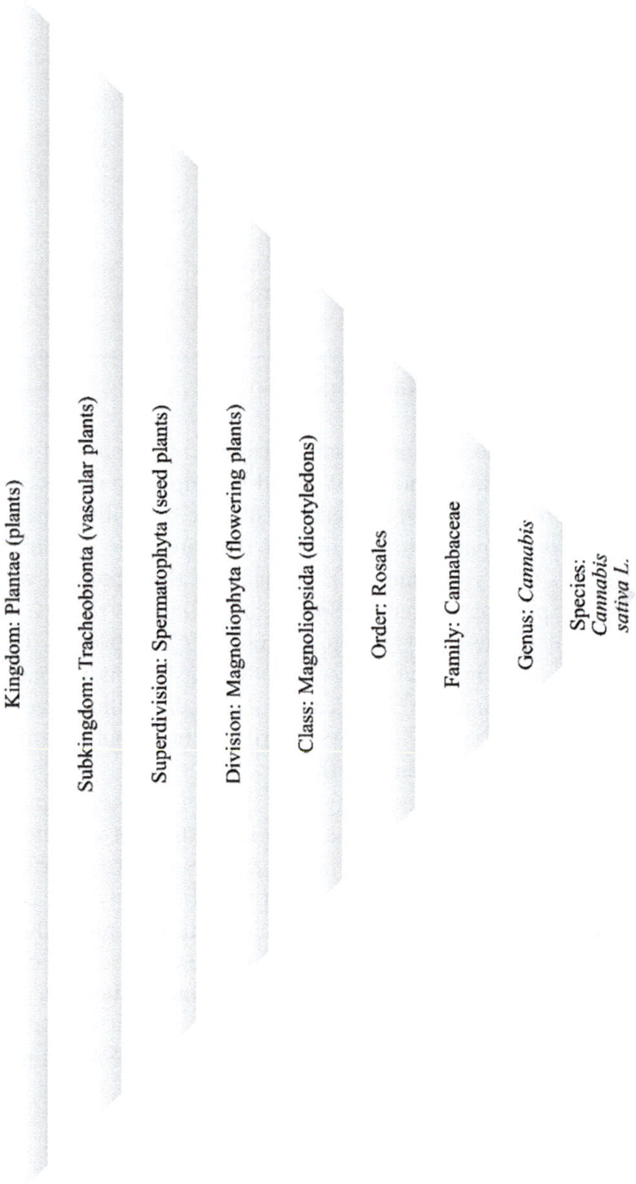

Kingdom: Plantae (plants)

Subkingdom: Tracheobionta (vascular plants)

Superdivision: Spermatophyta (seed plants)

Division: Magnoliophyta (flowering plants)

Class: Magnoliopsida (dicotyledons)

Order: Rosales

Family: Cannabaceae

Genus: *Cannabis*

Species: *Cannabis sativa L.*

Fig. 2.1 Linnaean classification of cannabis

products derived from other forms of cannabis (see Chap. 6 for more on cannabis regulatory issues).

"Marijuana" is a word that has been commonly used to refer to the cannabis plant for over a hundred years. This slang term, historically spelled "marihuana," came to the United States from Mexico in the early twentieth century, and though its linguistic origins are unclear, it has become the most well-known moniker for the cannabis plant [4]. Many advocates and industry professionals have pushed for a cultural shift to favor the word "cannabis" over "marijuana." In the first decades of the twentieth century, government regulators and sensationalist newspapers spread the idea that cannabis use was associated with violence and insanity and exploited racial tensions to gain support for anti-cannabis legislation, using the word "marijuana" to separate cannabis from its medicinal and industrial uses and stoke anti-immigrant tensions [5]. Although "marijuana" is not associated with racist connotations in modern American culture, many newer organizations, policies, and products use the word "cannabis" instead [6]. Other slang terms commonly used to describe the cannabis plant, many of which have been part of the American lexicon for decades, include "pot," "reefer," "dope," "Mary Jane," "weed," and "grass" [4].

Practice Tip
When counseling patients and communicating with other healthcare providers, use the word "cannabis." Using the scientific name helps to legitimize and professionalize cannabis medicine and will continue to dissociate cannabis from prohibition-era laws and attitudes. You're probably not referring to oxycodone/acetaminophen and methylphenidate tablets as "perks" and "smarties!"

2.2 Botanical Background

How does a plant come to be considered medicine? It's unlikely that early man was foraging around the edges of ancient lakes hoping to find the next great breakthrough in cancer treatment (a la Sean

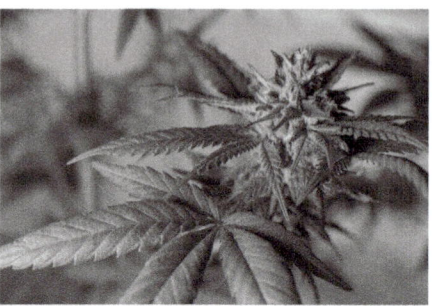

Fig. 2.2 *Cannabis sativa L.* leaves and flowers [8]

Connery in the movie *Medicine Man*). Cannabis appears to have originated in central and east Asia, where it was one of the earliest plants cultivated by man and valued for both its industrial uses and medicinal and psychoactive effects [7]. Like the more familiar opioids, evidence of medicinal cannabis use dates back thousands of years. Oral histories place the first medical use of cannabis in China around 2800 BC, with the first written evidence dating back to the first century AD [7]. In India, concoctions containing cannabis have been used socially and medicinally since around 1400 BC.

The cannabis plant is a remarkably hardy herbaceous weed due to a rapid (3–5 months) life cycle that enables it to flourish in many different environments [3]. Cannabis plants have a long stalk of fibers that may be used to make rope, cloth, and paper and distinct, serrated leaves with five to seven points (Fig. 2.2). The flowers of the female plant contain glandular hairs known as trichomes that secrete a resinous substance whose botanical purposes are likely to retain moisture and provide defense against herbivores, but which has long been valued by humans for the psychoactive substance it contains [3].

2.2.1   The Birds and the Bees and the Cannabis Plants

Cannabis is dioecious, meaning a single plant produces either male or female flowers. If you think we're getting just a *bit* in the weeds (pun intended, so sorry) talking about botanical reproduction in a book for healthcare providers, don't give up on this paragraph just yet. The reproductive characteristics of the cannabis plant significantly affect the production of chemicals of interest to humans. Female plants produce glandular trichomes that secrete resin, which has psychoactive properties in humans (the specific chemicals that have this effect are called "cannabinoids"—more about them shortly). All parts of the plant have been used throughout history for medicinal purposes, especially the flowers and seeds [9]. Seeds are produced only by the female plant after fertilization by a male plant. The resin produced by trichomes is also far more abundant in female plants. However, once fertilized, female plants spend energy producing seeds rather than resin, and therefore, cultivation of cannabis for medicinal or recreational purposes has long involved removing male plants (easily identified by their distinct morphology) prior to pollination, leading to seedless, resin-rich flowers on the female cannabis plant [3].

2.3   Phytochemicals: Cannabinoids, Terpenes, and Flavonoids, Oh My!

"Phytochemicals" are biologically active compounds originating in plants. These compounds are produced for myriad purposes, including defense against consumption by herbivores and regulation of growth, pollination, fertilization, and the surrounding soil [10]. Over 500 phytochemicals have been identified from the cannabis plant, and many have established or suspected effects on human physiology. Of most interest to a clinical audience are certain secondary metabolites (specialized compounds not directly involved in plant growth and reproduction), including cannabinoids, terpenes, and flavonoids. This chapter focuses on the botanical origins of these compounds, and Chap. 3 discusses their pharmacology.

2.3.1   Phytocannabinoids

Phytocannabinoids (i.e., cannabinoids originating in plants, distinct from endocannabinoids and synthetic cannabinoids) are a group of compounds identified by a common chemical structure that have a high affinity for cannabinoid receptors in humans. For a long time, cannabinoids were thought to be unique to the cannabis plant, but in the last decade or so, they have been found in several species of flower, liverwort, and fungus [11]. Cannabinoids are produced in the glandular trichomes present on the flowers of the female cannabis plant, with approximately 120 distinct cannabinoids identified so far [12]. The most abundant class of phytocannabinoids are those chemically similar to delta-9-tetrahydrocannabinol (commonly known as THC), which generally account for close to 20% of the total cannabinoid content in the plant. Other cannabinoid classes include cannabigerol-type (CBG), cannabidiol-type (CBD), cannabichromene-type (CBC), cannabinol-type, cannabitriol-type, cannabielsoin-type, cannabicyclol-type, and about 30 miscellaneous cannabinoids that don't fit neatly into any of the above classes [12].

The relative proportions of different cannabinoids may be affected by the environment in which they are grown. Cannabinoid production in trichomes is positively correlated with improved nutrition, light, soil, and time of harvest (e.g., before or after fertilization) [13]. If you've ever heard that THC levels in cannabis have been skyrocketing over the last half-century, improved control of these environmental factors is one reason why. Cannabinoids may have developed in plants as a defense mechanism (the sticky resin may have impaired herbivorous insects or at least given the very hungry caterpillar a strong desire for some Doritos and a nap) or to provide protection against ultraviolet light (exposure to which significantly increases cannabinoid production) [11].

2.3.2 Terpenes and Flavonoids

After cannabinoids, terpenes and terpenoids (oxygen-containing terpenes) are the next largest category of chemical compound found in the cannabis plant (over 100 have been identified) [14]. Unlike cannabinoids, terpenes are found in many plant types, and some of these are responsible for a plant's fragrance. Have you ever attended a rock concert, and suddenly you just *knew* that

Table 2.1 Commonly used terms in cannabis genomics

Word	Definition
Genotype	The genetic material in an individual plant
Phenotype	The observable traits that are the expression of the plant's genotype (leaf shape, color, etc.)
Chemotype	A plant's chemical composition (concentrations of phytochemicals, including cannabinoid and non-cannabinoid components). Also called *chemovar*
Strain	A specific variety of cannabis cultivated for particular traits (color, fragrance, pharmacological effects). Also called *cultivar*

Fig. 2.3 Terpenes are characterized by their chemical structure

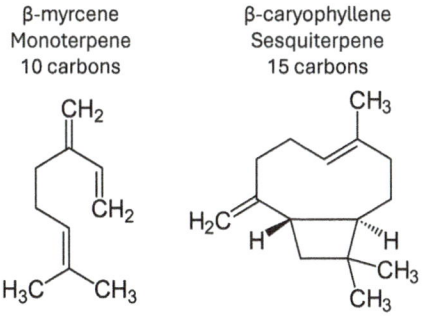

β-myrcene
Monoterpene
10 carbons

β-caryophyllene
Sesquiterpene
15 carbons

somewhere, someone in your general vicinity was smoking cannabis? That's terpenes. The familiar scents of many plants arise from distinct combinations of terpenes, a diverse group of volatile hydrocarbons that are the primary components of essential oils [15]. They are classified based on their chemical structure (Fig. 2.3); monoterpenes have 10 carbons, and sesquiterpenes have 15 carbons. In cannabis, common monoterpenes include α-pinene, β-myrcene, limonene, and linalool. The most common cannabis sesquiterpene is β-caryophyllene [16]. The botanical functions of terpenes include defense against herbivores and microorganisms and attracting pollinators and animals that can aid in seed dispersal. The low molecular weight, lipophilicity, and high vapor pressure of terpenes ensure that a plant's aroma can be detected even from a distance (like across the lawn at a rock concert). Flavonoids are antioxidants that protect the plant from reactive oxygen species produced under stressful environmental conditions like drought and excessive heat or cold [17]. Flavonoids also contribute to the plant's color, odor, and flavor. The antioxidant properties of flavonoids may be important to humans as well as plants, and there's a lot of interest in their therapeutic potential.

2.4   Exploring the Cannabis Genome

Like many cannabis-related topics, the genetic history of cannabis is not well understood and has been widely debated. The cannabis plant was first described only as *C. sativa* by Linnaeus in the eighteenth century. Since then, two other species (*C. indica* and *C. ruderalis*) have been proposed, rejected, and re-proposed. Genetic studies of cannabis plants grown in different geographic regions and with differing THC concentrations have not fully elucidated whether cannabis is a monotypic or polytypic plant species [18]. A lot has been written about the morphological differences between *C. indica* and *C. sativa* (*C. ruderalis* is considered a poor-quality plant, so it is not cultivated for human consumption). For instance, *C. sativa* is often characterized as having narrow leaves and *C. indica* as having broad leaves (Fig. 2.4) [19]. However, since all cannabis grown today is a hybrid of some sort, these classifications are not consistently applied. See Table 2.1 for some commonly used definitions related to cannabis genomics.

Sativa   Indica

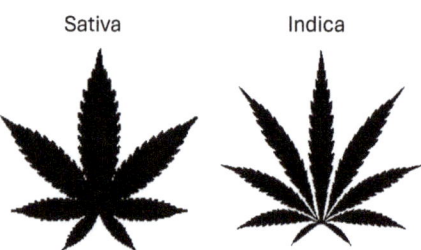

Fig. 2.4 The morphology of cannabis plants is often used to differentiate between proposed species

2.4.1   *C. sativa* Versus *C. indica*: What's in a Name (Part 2)?

It's common practice in the cannabis market to associate specific pharmacological effects with the broad botanical classifications of *C. sativa* and *C. indica*. For instance, *C. sativa* is often described as stimulating and energizing, whereas *C. indica* is described as relaxing or sedating. However, there is no evidence that an individual plant's pharmacological effects are related to its morphology. In fact, Ethan Russo, a distinguished cannabis researcher and physician, stated in an interview that "the sativa/indica distinction as commonly applied in the lay literature is total nonsense and an exercise in futility" [20].

Beyond *C. sativa* and *C. indica*, there is an urban dictionary's worth of creatively named cannabis strains, also commonly associated with specific chemotypes and pharmacological effects. However, unique cultivar names do not reliably represent distinct genotypes. Researchers in Canada genotyped 124 cannabis strains, comparing plants with the same name to the rest of the samples. They found that 35% of plants were more genetically similar to strains with different names than to strains with the same name [21]. Simply put, the "Northern Lights" strain from one dispensary, facility, or farm may not be the same as "Northern Lights" from another.

Practice Tip

How do you choose between "Malawi Gold" and "OG Kush"? Instead of recommending products based on strain name, teach patients to choose products based on their relative concentrations of cannabinoids (especially THC and CBD). Bonus tip: Get comfortable feeling a bit silly when having a discussion that includes questions about specific cannabis products or strains. If we as healthcare providers can get used to talking with patients about their bowel movements and sexual activity, we can take discussing "Gorilla Biscuit" and "Granddaddy Purple" in stride.

References

1. National Academies of Sciences, Engineering, and Medicine; Health and Medicine Division; Board on Population Health and Public Health Practice; Committee on the Health Effects of Marijuana: An Evidence Review and Research Agenda. The health effects of cannabis and cannabinoids: the current state of evidence and recommendations for research. Washington: National Academies Press; 2017.
2. Chaachouaya N, Azerouala A, Bencharkia B, Douirab A, Zidaneb L. Cannabis sativa L.: a review on traditional uses, botany, phytochemistry, and pharmacological aspects. Trad Integr Med. 2023;8(1):12407.
3. Merlin MD. Man and marijuana; some aspects of their ancient relationship. Rutherford: Fairleigh Dickinson University Press; 1972.
4. MacDonald T. A weed by any other name: culture, context, and the terminology shift from marijuana to cannabis. SSRN Electron J. 2023. https://papers.ssrn.com/sol3/papers.cfm?abstract_id=4322694.
5. Thompson M. The mysterious history of 'marijuana.' Code Switch. National Public Radio. 2013. https://www.npr.org/sections/codeswitch/2013/07/14/201981025/the-mysterious-history-of-marijuana.
6. Mikos RA, Kam CD. Has the "M" word been framed? Marijuana, cannabis, and public opinion. PLoS One. 2019;14(10):e0224289. https://doi.org/10.1371/journal.pone.0224289. PMID: 31671110; PMCID: PMC6822944.
7. Abel EL. Marihuana, the first twelve thousand years. New York: Plenum Press; 1980.
8. Hinterland E. Cannabis leaf [photograph]. Pixabay. 2020. https://pixabay.com/photos/marijuana-leaf-cannabis-leaf-5315557/.
9. Clarke RC, Merlin MD. Cannabis: evolution and ethnobotany. Berkeley: University of California Press; 2016.
10. Molyneux RJ, Lee ST, Gardner DR, Panter KE, James LF. Phytochemicals: the good, the bad and the ugly? Phytochemistry. 2007;68(22):2973–85.
11. Gülck T, Møller BL. Phytocannabinoids: origins and biosynthesis. Trends Plant Sci. 2020;25(10):985–1004.
12. Turner SE, Williams CM, Iversen L, Whalley BJ. Molecular pharmacology of phytocannabinoids. Phytocannabinoids. 2017;103:61–101.
13. Andre CM, Hausman JF, Guerriero G. Cannabis sativa: the plant of the thousand and one molecules. Front Plant Sci. 2016;7:19.
14. Radwan MM, Chandra S, Gul S, ElSohly MA. Cannabinoids, phenolics, terpenes and alkaloids of Cannabis. Molecules. 2021;26(9):2774.
15. Sommano SR, Chittasupho C, Ruksiriwanich W, Jantrawut P. The cannabis terpenes. Molecules. 2020;25(24):5792.
16. Booth JK, Bohlmann J. Terpenes in Cannabis sativa – from plant genome to humans. Plant Sci. 2019;284:67–72.

17. Dias MC, Pinto DCGA, Silva AMS. Plant flavonoids: chemical characteristics and biological activity. Molecules. 2021;26(17):5377. https://doi.org/10.3390/molecules26175377. PMID: 34500810; PMCID: PMC8434187.

18. Pollio A. The name of cannabis: a short guide for nonbotanists. Cannabis Cannabinoid Res. 2016;1(1):234–8. https://doi.org/10.1089/can.2016.0027. PMID: 28861494; PMCID: PMC5531363.

19. Punja ZK, Rodriguez G, Chen S. Assessing genetic diversity in Cannabis sativa using molecular approaches. In: Cannabis sativa L - botany and biotechnology. Cham: Springer; 2017. p. 395–418.

20. Piomelli D, Russo EB. The Cannabis sativa versus Cannabis indica debate: an interview with Ethan Russo, MD. Cannabis Cannabinoid Res. 2016;1(1):44–6. https://doi.org/10.1089/can.2015.29003.ebr.

21. Sawler J, Stout JM, Gardner KM, Hudson D, Vidmar J, Butler L, et al. The genetic structure of marijuana and hemp. PLoS ONE. 2015;10(8):e0133292.

Cannabinoid Pharmaceutical Science: Laying the Foundation for Cannabis Therapeutics

3

3.1 Lightning Round: Pharmacodynamics Review

Maybe you don't need to read this section because you remember everything you learned in pharmacy, medical, or nursing school. If that's the case, skip ahead to Sect. 3.3, where we get into the meat of this chapter. However, if, like many of us, a refresher on the basics couldn't hurt, read on. A middle-ground approach would be to review Table 3.1, which lists keywords and their definitions.

Cellular receptors are proteins that serve as targets for drugs and other ligands. When a ligand binds to its receptor on the surface of a cell, chemical signaling results in some effect or change inside the cell. Consider that many important activities occur inside the cell. When we administer a drug, it exists outside the cell—how does it cause intracellular changes without physically entering the cell itself? While a few classes of drugs physically cross lipid bilayer of the cell or bind to different types of proteins, most drugs exert their effects by binding to cell surface receptors and initiating a sequence of chemical messages like a very rapid and efficient game of "telephone." This chemical signaling results in the drug's pharmacological or pharmacodynamic effect (in lay language, "what the drug does to the body").

© The Author(s), under exclusive license to Springer Nature Switzerland AG 2025
L. Sera, C. Hempel-Sanderoff, *Cannabis Science and Therapeutics*, https://doi.org/10.1007/978-3-031-80352-9_3

Table 3.1 Pharmacology keywords and definitions

Keyword	Definition
Agonist/full agonist	A substance that binds to and activates a receptor, initiating a response
Allosteric modulator	A substance that binds to a receptor and changes the receptor's response to its endogenous ligand
Antagonist	A substance that binds to a receptor, preventing activation by its endogenous ligand
Binding affinity	The strength of the bond between a receptor and ligand (either endogenous ligand or drug)
Catalysis	Increased rate of chemical reaction
Enzyme	A protein that catalyzes a chemical reaction
Inverse agonist	A substance that binds to a receptor but initiates a pharmacological response that is opposite to its endogenous ligand
Ligand	A chemical substance that binds to a receptor
Partial agonist	A substance that binds to and activates a receptor, but produces less of a pharmacological response compared to a full agonist
Pharmacodynamics	The effects of a drug on the body
Pharmacokinetics	The effects of the body on a drug
Receptor	A protein that binds to a chemical substance (ligand) and initiates a chemical response inside a cell

3.1.1   Types of Drug-Receptor Interactions

Drugs are typically characterized as agonists, antagonists, partial agonists, or inverse agonists (see Fig. 3.1 for a graphical representation of this concept). An agonist is a drug that activates a receptor and leads to a biochemical response. Full agonists are often similar in structure to the receptor's endogenous ligand and have a similar effect. Partial agonists also lead to some effect after binding to a receptor, but there's a ceiling to that effect. A partial agonist given on top of a full agonist can mitigate the effect of the full agonist or prevent the full agonist from binding (that's why buprenorphine, a partial opioid receptor agonist, is used to treat addiction to heroin, a full agonist). Antagonists bind to receptors but do not activate them; instead, they block the binding site so that the receptor can't be activated by its endogenous ligand.

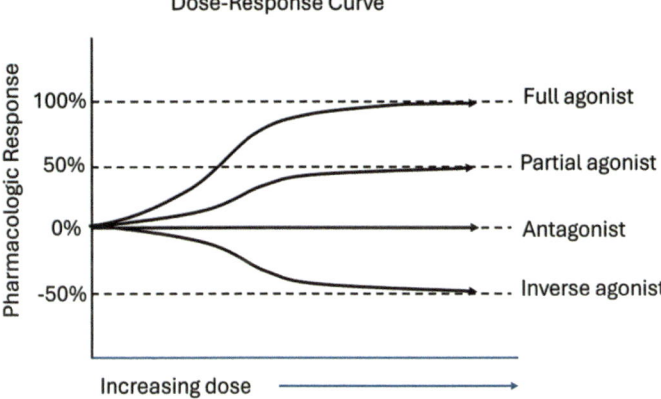

Fig. 3.1 A dose-response curve represents the relationship between medication dose and the magnitude of pharmacologic effect

Inverse agonists bind to the receptor, but instead of increasing receptor activity (a la agonists) or just sitting like a bump on a log (a la antagonists), inverse agonists actively decrease receptor activity. In practical terms, the effects of antagonists and inverse agonists appear to be very similar [1].

3.2   Lightning Round Part 2: Pharmacokinetics Review

If pharmacodynamics is "what the drug does to the body," then pharmacokinetics is "what the body does to the drug." What happens to the drug after it's administered? The short answer is absorption, distribution, metabolism, and elimination (referred to as "ADME" by generations of pharmacy school professors).

Absorption of a drug into the systemic circulation (i.e., the bloodstream, which carries the active drug molecule to its receptor target) can occur through the gut (oral administration), mucus membranes (transmucosal), skin (transdermal), muscle, subcutaneous layer, or lungs (inhalation) [2]. The amount of the drug initially administered that is available to bind with receptors after absorption is referred to as "bioavailability." Drugs injected intravenously have 100% bio-availability because no drug is lost in the absorption process (more accurately, there is no absorption process because the drug is administered directly into the systemic circulation). For some drugs, bio-availability is significantly affected by a phenomenon known as "first-pass metabolism," in which drugs undergo metabolism (usually in the liver) before reaching systemic circulation [3].

After a drug is delivered to the systemic circulation, *distribution* to the site of action occurs via the vasculature. While in the bloodstream, the drug may bind to proteins. Only free (i.e., unbound) drug is available for transport into other tissues where it can bind to its target and cause the intended pharmacodynamic effect. The physiochemical properties of drugs determine the location and extent of distribution in the body. Whether a compound is soluble in fat (lipophilic) or water (hydrophilic) is particularly important; lipophilic drugs more easily cross the lipid bilayer of the cell and the blood-brain barrier compared to hydrophilic compounds but must be transformed into more water-soluble compounds to be eliminated in the urine [4]. Distribution is also affected by an individual's water and fat composition (which is affected by lifestyle and health state).

Metabolism is the process of transforming a drug into a compound that is readily excreted from the body. After all, drugs can be helpful, but they're foreign to us, and the human body has some very complex machinery designed to efficiently remove molecular compounds that don't belong. Metabolism occurs in many different organ systems—the lungs, gut, and skin, for instance—but the workhorse of drug metabolism is the liver. Hepatic metabolism is described as either phase I or phase II. Phase I metabolism, also called biotransformation, renders lipophilic compounds more water-soluble to be excreted by the kidneys. Compounds are made more hydrophilic by adding or removing hydrogen and oxygen (oxidation, reduction, and hydrolysis). Often, this process renders the active compound inert, but sometimes, in the case of prodrugs, an inactive parent compound is transformed into an active metabolite [5]. Biotransformation is managed by the cytochrome P450 (CYP) system, a family of enzymes responsible for the phase I metabolism of many drugs.

To complicate matters, many drugs also inhibit or induce the activity of these CYP enzymes. In this way, the consumption of one drug may affect the metabolism of another, leading to drug-drug interactions and the potential for either toxicity or subtherapeutic effects (see Table 8.8 for a description of cannabis drug interactions). Phase II metabolism, known as conjugation, occurs when a polar (hydrophilic) molecule is attached to a drug to make it more water-soluble for excretion.

Elimination of drugs occurs primarily in the kidneys. The rate of clearance depends on both drug- and patient-related factors and influences drug dosing. Drugs may also be excreted via the feces, skin, and lungs. An important pharmacokinetic concept is the elimination half-life, which is the time required for the serum drug concentration to decrease by 50%. The rate of clearance and distribution profile both affect the elimination half-life.

3.3 Cannabinoid Pharmacology

Cannabinoid pharmacodynamic and pharmacokinetic effects depend on many factors and exhibit high variability between patients. This variability may be due to drug-related factors such as method of administration (i.e., inhaled versus oral versus oromucosal) and cannabis use patterns (i.e., dose, frequency, and administration technique) or patient-related factors such as age, body composition, genetics, and fed versus fasted state. This variability, combined with limited direct clinical research describing products available to patients in state cannabis markets, is why patients are often counseled to "start low and go slow" when determining the best dose and frequency to treat their symptoms. See Chap. 8 for much more discussion of dosing and monitoring.

3.3.1 Δ-9-tetrahydrocannabinol (THC) Pharmacodynamics

THC was the first phytocannabinoid identified in 1964 by Dr. Raphael Mechoulam, known by cannabis enthusiasts as the "father of cannabis research" [6]. THC and other cannabinoids exist in the cannabis plant as acids (e.g., THCA), which are decarboxylated to their neutral forms when heated (i.e., smoked or vaporized).

THC is classified as a partial agonist with high binding affinity at CB_1 receptors and CB_2 receptors and interacts directly or indirectly with a number of other receptors, including serotonin (5-HT) receptors, transient receptor potential (TRP) channels, GPCRs, and glycine receptors [7]. The pharmacodynamic effects of THC are associated primarily with the activation of CB_1 receptors in the CNS. As a high-affinity partial agonist, THC both attenuates the effects of full agonist endocannabinoids and blocks endocannabinoid receptor activation. It's unclear whether this or the resulting downregulation of endocannabinoids that occurs with chronic THC use has physiologic repercussions [8]. THC is the primary cannabinoid associated with psychoactive (i.e., altering mood, emotion, perception, or cognition) effects that result from downstream modulation of neurotransmitters like gamma-aminobutyric acid (GABA), dopamine, and glutamine [9]. That's why cannabis is associated with a risk of abuse and dependence (and the reason you're smelling cannabis at a rock concert). However, THC is also associated with many other physiologic effects (remember from Chap. 1 how widespread CB_1 receptors are throughout the body), including analgesia, antiemesis, appetite stimulation, cardiovascular effects, immunomodulation, and effects on reproductive systems. Synthetic THC (dronabinol) and a synthetic THC analog (nabilone) are approved by the US Food and Drug Administration (FDA) for the treatment of chemotherapy-induced nausea and vomiting. Nabiximols, a 1:1 THC/CBD transmucosal spray, is available outside the United States for muscle spasms associated with multiple sclerosis (Table 3.2 shows currently available forms of cannabis-based medicines).

Table 3.2 FDA-approved cannabinoid products

Generic drug name	Cannabinoid component	Formulation
Dronabinol	Synthetic THC	Oral capsule, solution
Nabilone	Synthetic THC analog	Oral capsule
CBD oil	Plant-derived CBD	Oral solution

3.3.2 THC Pharmacokinetics

Cannabinoids are highly lipophilic (fat-loving), a characteristic that has a significant effect on absorption via different routes of administration. The two most common administration methods are inhalation (smoking or vaporization) and oral (tinctures, edibles, and pharmaceutical preparations). After inhalation, THC reaches peak concentrations in 3–10 min and peak effect in 20–30 min [10]. The rapid absorption of THC contributes to its abuse liability. The bioavailability of inhaled cannabinoids depends on administration technique (inhalation volume, hold time, and the number, spacing, and duration of puffs) with reported bioavailability of around 30% (range 2–56%) [11]. Chronic users may have higher bioavailability than occasional users. In 1996, Adams and Martin reported that a dose of 2–22 mg smoked THC is required to produce a pharmacologic effect in humans [12]. Unlike inhalation, absorption of THC after oral administration is slow, with a much longer time to peak concentration and effect. After oral administration, THC undergoes extensive first-pass metabolism, resulting in low bioavailability (as low as 6%) and a significantly longer time to peak concentrations (C_{max}) compared to inhalation (60–120 min and as long as 4–6 h in some studies) [10].

THC is highly protein-bound in blood (95%), meaning that only about 5% of the bioavailable THC is free to interact with CB receptors [14]. As illustrated in Fig. 3.2, THC is rapidly distributed in high-perfusion tissues like the brain, liver, heart, lung, spleen, and placenta, resulting in a consequent decrease in plasma concentration [13]. Efflux pumps move THC quickly back out of the brain. Because cannabis is lipophilic, THC accumulates in adipose tissue, its long-term storage site, as both unaltered parent drug and metabolites [10]. THC persists in adipose tissue with chronic use for an extended period (weeks to months, depending on exposure). Adipose tissue releases THC back into circulation slowly, and THC plasma levels are not high enough to cause psychoactive effects—even though THC metabolites may be detectable in urine toxicology screening tests (see Chap. 5 for a more in-depth discussion of cannabis toxicology screening).

THC Pharmacokinetics

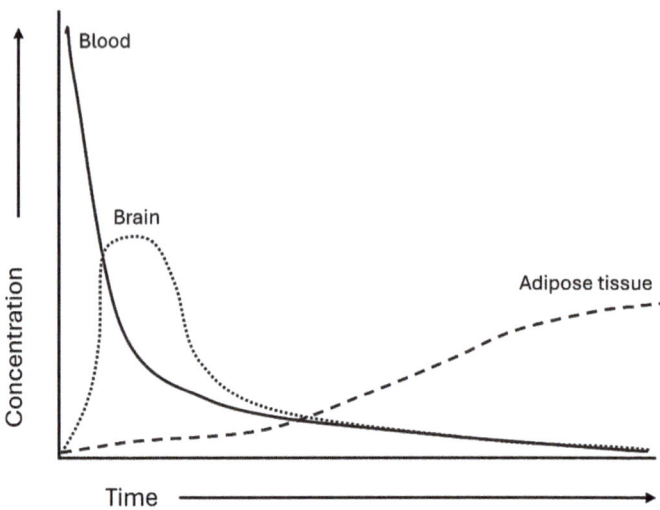

Fig. 3.2 THC is rapidly distributed to the brain and other high-perfusion tissues and accumulates in fat over time [13]

The metabolism of THC occurs primarily in the liver via biotransformation (phase I metabolism) by CYP enzymes 2C9, 2C19, and 3A4 (see Chap. 8 for a discussion of clinically significant drug interactions). The primary metabolites are 11-OH-THC (pronounced *11-hydroxy-THC*) and 11-COOH-THC (pronounced *11-carboxy-THC*). However, there are approximately 100 metabolites, such as ketones, aldehydes, carboxylic acids, and di- and trihydroxy compounds [11]. Additional metabolism occurs in other tissues, including the heart and lungs [10]. 11-OH-THC is equipotent to THC and has psychoactive effects. Much more 11-OH-THC is produced from oral administration compared to inhalation due to the effects of first-pass metabolism on orally ingested THC. 11-COOH-THC is the THC metabolite detected by urinary screening tests and is not associated with psychoactivity. The primary metabolites are further metabolized via glucuronidation (phase II metabolism) to increase hydrophilicity for excretion.

About 90% of THC is excreted within 5 days of use as hydroxylated or carboxylated metabolites. Most THC is excreted in the feces (65%) and urine (20%) [11]. The elimination half-life of THC is about 1 day in infrequent cannabis users and 5–10 days in frequent cannabis users [15]. In frequent users, the longer half-life is related to the slow release of THC from adipose tissue and significant enterohepatic recirculation [11].

Practice Tip
Counsel patients that a single dose of THC may be detectable in urine for about 3–5 days (but potentially up to a week or more). Frequent or daily users may have detectable levels of THC metabolites for weeks to months after last use. Become familiar with laws or policies in your state that provide protections or accommodations for registered medical cannabis patients (if these exist). Encourage your patients to find out if their workplace has policies in place to protect medical cannabis patients.

3.3.3 Cannabidiol (CBD) Pharmacodynamics

We don't know as much about the pharmacology of CBD as we do about THC. However, since CBD isn't associated with the same intoxicating psychoactive effects and abuse potential as THC, there is a lot of interest in illuminating its therapeutic potential. CBD has reported agonist, inverse agonist, or antagonist activity at many different types of receptors but (perhaps surprisingly) has a low affinity for both CB_1 and CB_2 receptors [16]. Instead of activating CB receptors, CBD may act as a weak antagonist or as an allosteric modulator at CB receptors. In cell-based studies, CBD has been shown to interact with glycine receptors, GABA receptors, 5-HT receptors, nicotinic receptors, TRP channels, voltage-gated ion channels, nuclear receptors, and enzymes [16]. CBD inhibits FAAH, the enzyme that breaks down anandamide. CBD has neuroprotective, immunomodulating, and anti-inflammatory properties; it is an effective anticonvulsant, and it shows promise as an anxiolytic and antipsychotic agent (see Chap. 4 for a more in-depth discussion of the medical literature) [17]. CBD oil is FDA-approved to treat some severe seizure disorders that primarily affect children.

3.3.4   CBD Pharmacokinetics

Like THC, CBD bioavailability varies between different modes of administration, and study results show a wide range. When inhaled, CBD has a bioavailability of around 30% (range 11–45%) and a bioavailability when taken orally of around 15% (range 6–21%) [10]. CBD undergoes first-pass metabolism. CBD is also highly protein-bound (>95%) and readily distributed to highly vascularized tissues. CBD undergoes hepatic phase I metabolism by CYP2C19 and CYP3A4 to active and inactive metabolites prior to glucuronidation to increase hydrophilicity for excretion. CBD is also a substrate for CYP1A2, CYP2C9, and CYP2D6 [17]. The elimination half-life of CBD is approximately 18–32 h [18].

3.4   The Pharmacology of Selected Minor Cannabinoids

There's a lot of interest in the cannabis research community in minor cannabinoids and terpenes, with the NIH providing funding for both preclinical and clinical research in this area. One reason is that many of the minor cannabinoids and terpenes may have therapeutic value but are not associated with intoxicating effects and, therefore, may provide an alternative to THC.

Cannabinol (*CBN*) is a THC metabolite produced by oxidation. CBN is an agonist at both CB_1 and CB_2 receptors, with much lower affinity than THC [19]. CBN also acts as an agonist at TRPs, ion channels associated with heat and cold sensation (these are the receptors activated by capsaicin—a chemical found in chili peppers that makes you really regret rubbing your eyes after making salsa). Several animal studies have demonstrated analgesic, anti-inflammatory, and orexigenic effects. A cannabinol cream is being studied to treat a rare skin disease called epidermolysis bullosa, demonstrating superior anti-itch activity compared to control in phase II trials (phase II trials are small human clinical trials evaluating the effect of a drug in subjects with a particular disease or condition) [20].

Cannabichromene (*CBC*) is a stereoisomer of CBD (the same chemical formula with the atoms in a different spatial arrangement). It is produced at very low levels in most cannabis cultivars (less than 1%), making extraction difficult [21]. CBC is a selective CB_2 receptor agonist and may increase endocannabinoid concentrations by inhibiting the activity of the 2-AG hydrolyzing enzyme monoacylglycerol lipase [22]. CBC is an agonist at TRP channels and PPARs (these receptors are most commonly recognized by clinicians as the targets for the hypolipidemic fibrates and the antidiabetic thiazolidinediones). Preclinical studies (both in vitro and in vivo) indicate that CBC may have therapeutic potential as an anti-inflammatory agent. CBC has also been shown in animal models to have anticonvulsant activity similar to CBD as well as analgesic activity [23]. CBC does not produce intoxicating effects, making it an attractive candidate as a therapeutic modality.

Cannabigerol (*CBG*) accounts for only 10% of cannabinoid content in the cannabis plant, although its precursor (cannabigerolic acid or CBGA) is a precursor to both THC and CBD acids via enzymatic activity [24]. CBG is thought to be a weak partial agonist at both CB_1 and CB_2 receptors with affinity 5–27 times less than that of THC (though some studies indicate negligible binding affinity) [25]. CBG has activity comparable to CBD at TRP channels, is a 5-HT receptor antagonist, and, uniquely among the cannabinoids (as far as we know), is a potent α-2 adrenergic receptor agonist (α-2 agonists mimic the effects of epinephrine and norepinephrine in the body) [26]. CBG undergoes phase I metabolism in the liver via CYP3A4 and CYP2C9. CBG is not psychoactive and, like other minor cannabinoids, has been shown to have anti-inflammatory and antioxidant effects in preclinical studies. CBG has also shown in vitro anti-tumor activity against some cancer cell lines [27].

3.5   The Entourage Effect

When Raphael Mechoulam's research team was studying the pharmacology of cannabinoid receptors in the 1990s, they found that endocannabinoid activity at CB_1 receptors was augmented by the presence of organic compounds that had no direct effect on the receptor. They extrapolated this finding to hypothesize that the many chemical compounds in the cannabis plant would produce a stronger pharmacologic effect than the isolated components. They dubbed this the "entourage effect" [28]. This is an incredibly popular theory despite the lack of supporting evidence, perhaps because it implies the added benefit of natural or botanical medicine compared to pharmaceuticals.

Many components of the cannabis plant have physiological effects, including cannabinoids and terpenes. However, preclinical and clinical studies have not yet provided a robust answer to the question of whether whole-plant or full-spectrum cannabis products are more effective than cannabinoid isolates. In two cell-based studies, researchers evaluated the effect of six common terpenes on CB receptors. In both studies, the terpenes (on their own or in combination) didn't activate the receptors directly or have any effect on the activation of CB receptors by THC [29, 30]. One area of interest is the attenuating effect of CBD on the negative psychoactive effects of THC, such as anxiety, paranoia, and toxic psychosis. Published clinical trials that compare whole-plant or full-spectrum products to cannabinoid isolates are generally small with conflicting results [28]. Though the absence of evidence is not evidence of absence, for now, the entourage effect should be considered a scientific possibility rather than an evidence-based approach to cannabis medicine.

3.6   Cannabis Toxicity

Cannabis products come in a variety of formulations. What most people probably picture when hearing the phrase "medical cannabis" is a joint (i.e., cannabis cigarette) or perhaps the dried flower itself. However, there are many other formulations and routes of administration. The dried flower may be ground up and rolled into joints or smoked in pipes or bongs (water pipes). The THC content in most cannabis cultivated today is around 20% (a far cry from the 2% THC in the cannabis you'd find at a Bob Dylan concert in the 1980s). The cannabinoids can be extracted from the plant by soaking the plant in a solvent and applying heat and/or pressure to the resulting mixture until the solvent evaporates and leaves behind an oil, wax, or hard solid with a THC concentration of 70–90%. These concentrates, called hash, wax, shatter, or oil (depending on the extraction process used), can be ingested or inhaled. Cannabis can also be infused into baked goods, candies, and beverages. Chapter 8 discusses dosing and administration considerations with various products and formulations.

3.6.1 Misadventures and Accidental Ingestions

With the legalization of non-medical (i.e., recreational or "adult-use") cannabis in many states, the variety of formulations and increasing THC concentrations may lead to misadventures, accidental ingestion by children, and the resulting potential for toxicity. Accidental overuse in adults is most often related to ingestion of edible products; the delayed onset of action may lead inexperienced users to re-dose prematurely. In teens and adults, acute cannabis toxicity typically presents as dysphoria, anxiety, or agitation [31]. Patients with underlying pulmonary or cardiovascular disease may have additional risks for exacerbation. Toxicity is more serious in children (who might accidentally ingest cannabis-containing edible products that appear to be innocuous), who may present with lethargy, decreased muscle coordination, seizures, or, in the most critical cases, coma [32]. Cannabis is not associated with fatal overdose directly; however, fatalities may occur due to accidents resulting from altered cognition. Due to the stigma associated with cannabis use, patients may be reluctant to admit to cannabis use in the healthcare setting, leading to unnecessary and costly diagnostic tests and procedures.

   Long-term, regular use of cannabis is increasingly being associated with a cyclic vomiting condition called cannabis hyperemesis syndrome (CHS). Symptoms of CHS include intermittent periods of severe nausea, vomiting, and abdominal pain in the setting of frequent (often daily) cannabis use [33]. Individuals also often experience compulsive hot water bathing, which provides temporary relief. This condition is thought to be due to overstimulation of cannabinoid receptors in the brain and the gut and possibly associated with cannabinoid effects on TRP receptors [34]. Treatment includes cessation of cannabis use and supportive therapy.

3.6.2   Illicit Synthetic Cannabinoids

Researchers have been synthesizing cannabinoids for decades: first, to study the physiological effects of THC in the 1960s and then to develop the pharmaceutical agents dronabinol and nabilone, which were approved in the 1980s to treat chemotherapy-induced nausea and vomiting. However, in the 1990s, an investigator with good intentions but regrettably poor foresight synthesized a synthetic THC compound and published multiple papers and a book about it—including the formula—upon which eager, less-well-intentioned chemists pounced for their own commercial gain [35].

Synthetic cannabinoids do not resemble natural cannabinoids, including THC, chemically speaking. However, they bind CB_1 receptors with a much higher affinity than THC and act as full agonists (unlike THC, which is a partial agonist). These compounds are sprayed on non-cannabis plant material and sold in gas stations, convenience stores, head shops, and online. There is no medical benefit associated with these illicit synthetic cannabinoids, and many have been deemed Schedule I substances (i.e., no currently accepted medical use and a high likelihood of abuse). Illicit synthetic cannabinoids have a higher risk of toxicity compared to natural cannabinoids and have been associated with nausea, vomiting, agitation, tachycardia, bradycardia, hypertension, hypotension, seizures, acute kidney injury, lethargy, tachypnea, new-onset psychosis, and myocardial infarction [36]. In fact, synthetic cannabinoids might precipitate the zombie apocalypse; first responders to a mass intoxication event in Brooklyn in 2016 reported that casualties exhibited "zombie-like" behavior (groaning, lethargic, blank stare, and slow, purposeless limb movements) [37].

3.7   A Few Words About Cannabinoid Chemistry

For compounds with such distinct pharmacology, you may be surprised to learn that THC and CBD have almost identical chemical structures (Fig. 3.3). The only difference is that THC has a closed ring, while CBD has an open ring—and that one difference completely changes the pharmacodynamics of the molecule. Seeing how similar these compounds are, you might not be surprised to find out that it is not that difficult to use chemistry to transform CBD into THC. You might have seen or heard about a kind of THC being sold in gas stations and convenience stores—this is Δ-8-THC. This isomer of Δ-9-THC, in which a carbon-carbon double bond is shifted from the 9-position in an aromatic ring to the 8-position in an aromatic ring, exists in minute quantities in the cannabis plant. However, enterprising chemists found that loads of Δ-8-THC can be created by boiling CBD in acid. Is this legal? It's complicated.

When the Agriculture Improvement Act of 2018 (also known as the Farm Bill) removed hemp (i.e., cannabis plants containing less than 0.3% THC) from the definition of "marijuana" in the

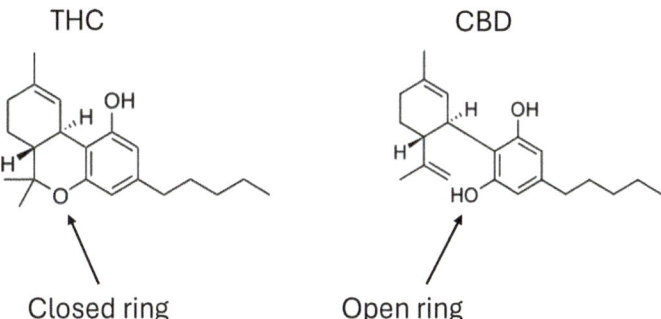

Fig. 3.3   The chemical structures of THC and CBD

CSA, making it legal to grow in the United States, hemp-derived CBD products began flooding the market (unregulated by the FDA) in the form of creams and lip balms and supplements. Because hemp that is grown in accordance with federal regulations is legal in the United States, psychoactive THC isomers, precursors, and derivatives (including Δ-8-THC, Δ-10-THC, THC-O, and others) manufactured from hemp-derived CBD are also legal—at least for now. An amendment added to the 2024 Farm Bill draft closes the loophole that allows these products to be sold legally.

3.8   From Plant to Product: Cannabinoid Drug Development

The modern drug development process in the United States traditionally starts with the identification of a biochemical pathway associated with a disease process that could be the target of a new pharmaceutical agent. Then, a molecule that meets the requirements is identified and tested in human cells (in vitro studies) and in animals (in vivo studies). Compounds that appear to be effective are formulated into medications for administration in humans during a series of clinical trials to evaluate the drug's safety and effectiveness. The FDA reviews all the data and decides whether the drug is approved and can be sold to patients. But what about botanical products? Plants are complex organisms that contain hundreds of chemicals, many of which are biologically active. This is entirely at odds with traditional drug development, which takes a single molecule and formulates a delivery vehicle to get the molecule to its specific biological target. The only plant-derived FDA-approved cannabinoid product currently available in the United States is CBD oil, which is a single cannabinoid extract from cannabis. There is published guidance for the pharmaceutical industry regarding the development of botanicals for FDA approval [38]. Some issues that manufacturers of cannabis products will have to contend with include therapeutic consistency (challenging considering the variability between plants), good manufacturing and cultivation practices, and defining the pharmacology of a formulation with multiple active compounds.

References

1. Berg KA, Clarke WP. Making sense of pharmacology: inverse agonism and functional selectivity. Int J Neuropsychopharmacol. 2018;21(10):962–77. https://doi.org/10.1093/ijnp/pyy071. PMID: 30085126; PMCID: PMC6165953.
2. Sera LC, Mcpherson ML. Pharmacokinetics and pharmacodynamic changes associated with aging and implications for drug therapy. Clin Geriatr Med. 2012;28(2):273–86. https://doi.org/10.1016/j.cger.2012.01.007.
3. Herman TF, Santos C. First-pass effect. In: StatPearls. Treasure Island: StatPearls Publishing; 2024. https://www.ncbi.nlm.nih.gov/books/NBK551679/.
4. Onetto AJ, Sharif S. Drug distribution. In: StatPearls. Treasure Island: StatPearls Publishing; 2024. https://www.ncbi.nlm.nih.gov/books/NBK567736/.
5. Susa ST, Hussain A, Preuss CV. Drug metabolism. In: StatPearls. Treasure Island: StatPearls Publishing; 2024. https://www.ncbi.nlm.nih.gov/books/NBK442023/.
6. Raphael Mechoulam WA. Father of Cannabis Research, dies at 92. New York Times. 2023. https://www.nytimes.com/2023/03/22/science/raphael-mechoulam-dead.html. Accessed 27 August 2024.
7. Ligresti A, De Petrocellis L, Di Marzo V. From phytocannabinoids to cannabinoid receptors and endocannabinoids: pleiotropic physiological and pathological roles through complex pharmacology. Physiol Rev. 2016;96(4):1593–659. https://doi.org/10.1152/physrev.00002.2016.
8. Haney M. Cannabis use and the endocannabinoid system: a clinical perspective. Am J Psychiatry. 2022;179(1):21–5. https://doi.org/10.1176/appi.ajp.2021.21111138.
9. Sera L, Hempel-Sanderoff C. Cannabis science and therapeutics: an overview for clinicians. J Clin Pharmacol. 2024;64(5):499–513. https://doi.org/10.1002/jcph.2400. Epub 2024 Jan 17.
10. Grotenhermen F. Pharmacokinetics and pharmacodynamics of cannabinoids. Clin Pharmacokinet. 2003;42(4):327–60.
11. Huestis MA. Human cannabinoid pharmacokinetics. Chem Biodivers. 2007;4(8):1770–804.
12. Adams IB, Martin BR. Cannabis: pharmacology and toxicology in animals and humans. Addiction. 1996;91(11):1585–614.
13. Ashton CH. Pharmacology and effects of cannabis: a brief review. Br J Psychiatry. 2001;178(2):101–6.
14. Hunt CA, Jones RT. Tolerance and disposition of tetrahydrocannabinol in man. J Pharmacol Exp Ther. 1980;215(1):35–44.
15. Smith-Kielland A, Skuterud B, Mørland J. Urinary excretion of 11-nor-9-carboxy-delta9-tetrahydrocannabinol and cannabinoids in frequent and

infrequent drug users. J Anal Toxicol. 1999;23(5):323–32. https://doi.org/10.1093/jat/23.5.323.

16. Castillo-Arellano J, Canseco-Alba A, Cutler SJ, León F. The polypharmacological effects of cannabidiol. Molecules. 2023;28(7):3271.

17. Zendulka O, Dovrtělová G, Nosková K, Turjap M, Šulcová A, Hanuš L, Juřica J. Cannabinoids and cytochrome P450 interactions. Curr Drug Metab. 2016;17(3):206–26. https://doi.org/10.2174/138920021766615121014205l.

18. Chayasirisobhon S. Mechanisms of action and pharmacokinetics of cannabis. Perm J. 2020;25(1):1–3.

19. Maioli C, Mattoteia D, Amin HIM, Minassi A, Caprioglio D. Cannabinol: history, syntheses, and biological profile of the greatest "minor" cannabinoid. Plants. 2022;11(21):2896. https://doi.org/10.3390/plants11212896. PMID: 36365350; PMCID: PMC9658060.

20. INM-755 Cannabinol (CBN) cream. InMed Pharmaceuticals. [Internet]. 2024. https://www.inmedpharma.com/pharmaceutical/inm-755-for-epidermolysis-bullosa/. Accessed 27 August 2024.

21. DeLong GT, Wolf CE, Poklis A, Lichtman AH. Pharmacological evaluation of the natural constituent of Cannabis sativa, cannabichromene and its modulation by Δ(9)-tetrahydrocannabinol. Drug Alcohol Depend. 2010;112(1-2):126–33. https://doi.org/10.1016/j.drugalcdep.2010.05.019. PMID: 20619971; PMCID: PMC2967639.

22. Udoh M, Santiago M, Devenish S, McGregor IS, Connor M. Cannabichromene is a cannabinoid CB2 receptor agonist. Br J Pharmacol. 2019;176(23):4537–47. https://doi.org/10.1111/bph.14815. Epub 2019 Nov 21. PMID: 31368508; PMCID: PMC6932936.

23. Sepulveda DE, Vrana KE, Kellogg JJ, Bisanz JE, Desai D, Graziane NM, et al. The potential of cannabichromene (CBC) as a therapeutic agent. J Pharmacol Exp Ther. 2024;391(2):206–13.

24. Jastrząb A, Jarocka-Karpowicz I, Skrzydlewska E. The origin and biomedical relevance of cannabigerol. Int J Mol Sci. 2022;23(14):7929. https://doi.org/10.3390/ijms23147929. PMID: 35887277; PMCID: PMC9322760.

25. Nachnani R, Raup-Konsavage WM, Vrana KE. The pharmacological case for cannabigerol. J Pharmacol Exp Ther. 2021;376(2):204–12.

26. Cascio MG, Gauson LA, Stevenson LA, Ross RA, Pertwee RG. Evidence that the plant cannabinoid cannabigerol is a highly potent alpha2-adrenoceptor agonist and moderately potent 5HT1A receptor antagonist. Br J Pharmacol. 2010;159(1):129–41. https://doi.org/10.1111/j.1476-5381.2009.00515.x. Epub 2009 Dec 4. PMID: 20002104; PMCID: PMC2823359.

27. Calapai F, Cardia L, Esposito E, Ammendolia I, Mondello C, Lo Giudice R, Gangemi S, Calapai G, Mannucci C. Pharmacological aspects and biological effects of cannabigerol and its synthetic derivatives. Evid Based Complement Alternat Med. 2022;2022:3336516. https://doi.org/10.1155/2022/3336516.

28. Simei JLQ, Souza JDR, Lisboa JR, Campos AC, Guimarães FS, Zuardi A, et al. Does the "entourage effect" in cannabinoids exist? A narrative scoping review. Cannabis Cannabinoid Res. 2023;9(5):1202–16.

29. Santiago M, Sachdev S, Arnold JC, Mcgregor IS, Connor M. Absence of entourage: terpenoids commonly found in Cannabis sativa do not modulate the functional activity of Δ9-THC at human CB1 and CB2 receptors. Cannabis Cannabinoid Res. 2019;4(3):165–76. https://doi.org/10.1089/can.2019.0016.

30. Heblinski M, Santiago M, Fletcher C, et al. Terpenoids commonly found in Cannabis sativa do not modulate the actions of phytocannabinoids or endocannabinoids on TRPA1 and TRPV1 channels. Cannabis Cannabinoid Res. 2020;5(4):305–17. https://doi.org/10.1089/can.2019.0099.

31. Noble MJ, Hedberg K, Hendrickson RG. Acute cannabis toxicity. Clin Toxicol. 2019;57(8):735–42.

32. Kelly BF, Nappe TM. Cannabinoid toxicity. In: StatPearls. Treasure Island: StatPearls Publishing; 2024. https://www.ncbi.nlm.nih.gov/books/NBK482175/.

33. Lathrop JR, Rosen SN, Heitkemper MM, Buchanan DT. Cyclic vomiting syndrome and cannabis hyperemesis syndrome: the state of the science. Gastroenterol Nurs. 2023;46(3):208–24.

34. Cue L, Chu F, Cascella M. Cannabinoid hyperemesis syndrome. In: StatPearls. Treasure Island: StatPearls Publishing; 2024. https://www.ncbi.nlm.nih.gov/books/NBK549915/.

35. McCoy T. How this chemist unwittingly helped spawn the synthetic drug industry. The Washington Post. 2015. https://www.washingtonpost.com/local/social-issues/how-a-chemist-unwittingly-helped-spawn-the-synthetic-drug-epidemic/2015/08/09/94454824-3633-11e5-9739-170df8af8eb9_story.html. Accessed 27 August 2024.

36. Leonard J. Synthetic cannabinoids: an undetectable and uncomfortable high. Baltimore: University of Maryland School of Pharmacy; 2018.

37. Adams AJ, Banister SD, Irizarry L, Trecki J, Schwartz M, Gerona R. "Zombie" outbreak caused by the synthetic cannabinoid AMB-FUBINACA in New York. N Engl J Med. 2017;376(3):235–42. https://doi.org/10.1056/NEJMoa1610300.

38. Center for Drug Evaluation and Research. Botanical drug development: guidance for industry [Internet]. U.S. Food and Drug Administration. 2016. https://www.fda.gov/regulatory-information/search-fda-guidance-documents/botanical-drug-development-guidance-industry. Accessed 27 August 2024.

Clinical Uses of Cannabinoids: What Does the Evidence Say?

4

4.1 Brief Overview of the Clinical Evidence Landscape

One of the most common refrains from clinicians regarding medical cannabis is the perception of a lack of evidence to guide understanding of safety and efficacy. The current federal legal status of cannabis in the United States (designated a Schedule I drug under the Controlled Substances Act or CSA) has severely limited high-quality research over the past decades (see Chap. 6 for a more in-depth overview of the cannabis regulatory landscape). In the past 10 years, many studies have been published exploring the therapeutic uses of cannabinoids. However, clinicians should critically evaluate all such studies utilizing a keen understanding of study design, methodology, and the risk of bias.

4.2 The Pyramid of Evidence and the Influence of Study Designs

Applying an evidence-based approach to the cannabis medical literature involves a review of the hierarchy of study design and utility. The typical "gold standard" randomized controlled trials (RCTs) are fraught with challenges, including lack of standardization of cannabis plants and products, limited research settings

© The Author(s), under exclusive license to Springer Nature Switzerland AG 2025
L. Sera, C. Hempel-Sanderoff, *Cannabis Science and Therapeutics*,
https://doi.org/10.1007/978-3-031-80352-9_4

due to Schedule I legal status in the United States, and difficulty blinding due to the psychoactivity of THC. Additionally, there are a limited number of approved cannabis suppliers for United States-based research, which reduces the generalizability of study findings (because it's nearly impossible to do reproducible research on the products that patients are actually obtaining at dispensaries and other cannabis retailers). Many clinical studies involving cannabis are observational or quasi-experimental (i.e., nonrandomized). Interpreting and applying results from myriad study designs of varying quality remains a barrier for clinicians seeking to understand the usefulness of cannabis-based medicines and dispensary products, which are not standardized or regulated. Cannabis studies often have poor generalizability and low external validity due to this lack of standardization (Fig. 4.1).

One way to improve the value of cannabis research is through "phase IV" studies (so named because they follow the three phases of clinical trials in the drug development pathway). These

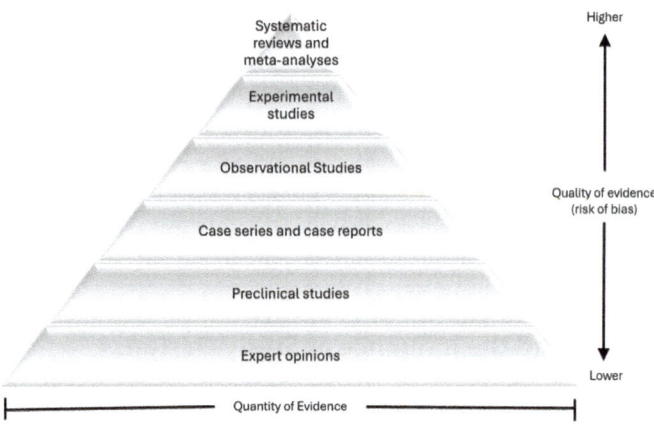

Fig. 4.1 Systematic reviews and meta-analyses are the highest quality evidence, followed by experimental studies (i.e., randomized controlled trials), observational studies (cohort, case-control, and cross-sectional), case series and case reports, preclinical studies (animal- and cell-based), and expert opinion. There is a much higher quantity of low-quality evidence (high risk of bias), compared to high-quality evidence (lower risk of bias) [1]

studies examine the real-world effects of medications by evaluating post-marketing data regarding the effects of pharmaceuticals and other approved medical treatments [2]. Whereas phase I, II, and III clinical trials provide information regarding how a new drug interacts with a human being or a select population, phase IV studies examine the effects of the drug in a broader population and more natural setting. In contrast to RCTs, phase IV studies are observational, not experimental. The purpose of these studies is to counter the lack of external validity (i.e., generalizability) of RCTs, which often exclude populations that may use the treatment in the "real world" or which are conducted under circumstances that do not mirror the true patient experience (i.e., more frequent or more in-depth clinical encounters). These studies may help elucidate the true effects of a new medication on the general public in a natural setting. These studies offer a complementary and valuable perspective when combined with evidence from RCTs and are increasingly used to assess the effects of the ever-growing number of cannabis products and formulations on the market.

4.3   Much Ado About Cannabis: What Are Patients Looking For?

It's often said that access to cannabis has outpaced evidence, and we discuss the cannabis regulatory landscape in detail in Chap. 6. A question as important as "*how* did this happen?" is "*why* did this happen?" What are patients looking for that they aren't finding in the bottles stocking pharmacy shelves? For what conditions are patients seeking cannabis as a therapeutic modality, and how does the evidence base line up with patients' hopes and expectations?

In the United States, the most common conditions for which adults report using medical cannabis are chronic pain, anxiety, insomnia, and depression [3]. Chronic pain is the most cited qualifying condition (i.e., a condition for which a patient can be legally certified to use medical cannabis) in US jurisdictions that have a legal medical cannabis program [4]. In 2024, the FDA released a report in support of rescheduling in which regulators concluded that on the basis of currently available, credible scientific evidence, cannabis can be said to have a "currently accepted medical use" (a requirement for removal from Schedule I under the CSA) for pain, nausea and vomiting, and anorexia related to a medical condition [5]. Previously, an exhaustive systematic review published in 2017 by the National Academies of Sciences, Engineering, and Medicine (NASEM) classified conditions as having conclusive, substantial, limited, or no/insufficient clinical evidence supporting cannabis use (Table 4.1) [7]. Over the past decade, an increasing number of patients have been certified to use medical cannabis with qualifying conditions classified as having limited or insufficient evidence for use, in addition to conditions recorded as vaguely such as "other" and "psychiatric condition" [4]. Additionally, the use of hemp-derived CBD, most commonly for anxiety, insomnia, and pain, has climbed rapidly since the production of hemp was legalized in the 2018 Farm Bill,

Table 4.1 Effectiveness of cannabinoids for selected medical conditions [4, 6]

Level of evidence	Description	Medical conditions
Conclusive	• Strong evidence from RCTs and many good-quality studies • Very few or no credible opposing findings	• Chemotherapy-induced nausea and vomiting • Seizures associated with Lennox-Gastaut and Dravet syndromes
Substantial	• Strong evidence from several good-quality studies • Very few or no credible opposing findings	• Chronic pain • Spasticity associated with multiple sclerosis
Moderate	• Several findings from good- to fair-quality studies • Very few or no credible opposing findings	• Insomnia

(continued)

Table 4.1   (continued)

Level of evidence	Description	Medical conditions
Limited	• Supportive findings from fair-quality studies • Mixed findings, with most favoring effectiveness	• HIV/AIDS-associated anorexia/cachexia • Symptoms associated with Tourette's syndrome, social anxiety disorder, and post-traumatic stress disorder (PTSD)
None	• Mixed findings or a single poor-quality study or no clinical studies have been conducted	• Anorexia nervosa • Cancer • Cancer-associated anorexia/cachexia • Dystonia • Schizophrenia • Spasticity associated with spinal cord injury • Substance use disorders • Symptoms associated with Huntington's disease, amyotrophic lateral sclerosis, and Parkinson's disease

even though there is scant evidence supporting the use of CBD for these indications [8].

4.4   The Evidence Base for Selected Medical Conditions

A growing body of evidence is helping to elucidate the role of cannabis and cannabinoids in medical management. This section summarizes the evidence base for selected symptoms and conditions.

4.4.1   Chronic Non-cancer Pain

The location of CB receptors in key areas of the central and peripheral nervous system suggests the potential usefulness of endo- and phytocannabinoids in the modulation of nociception and production of analgesic effects [9]. Over the past 20 years, both synthetic and whole-plant cannabis formulations have been studied on different types of chronic, non-cancer pain, including neuropathic and inflammatory pain. The most robust evidence indicates that oral preparations of balanced THC and CBD in equal ratios (1:1) may provide pain reductions greater than 30% (i.e., clinically significant) in several conditions, including painful spasticity in multiple sclerosis, chronic neuropathic pain, inflammatory arthritis pain, and generalized chronic pain [10]. Smaller studies have evaluated different preparations, including inhaled THC and topical CBD, with mixed results [11, 12]. A large observational, long-term longitudinal study of patients with chronic pain demonstrated reduced pain scores and improved quality of life (QOL) with the use of various forms of medical cannabis, with trends toward greater improvement over longer durations of use. However, a large proportion of the participants reported smoking dried herbal cannabis, while others were using cannabis oils or other combinations from local dispensaries, limiting the study's generalizability [12].

In the United States and the world, the medical community is grappling with two epidemics: chronic pain and opioid misuse and abuse. The opioid crisis necessitates the exploration of alternative treatments for chronic pain. The ECS and its widespread regulation of neurotransmitters, nerve conduction, and nociception is an attractive therapeutic target for developing a new generation of analgesic treatments. There are many barriers to conducting robust, gold standard clinical trials of cannabis for chronic pain, including regulatory, supply, and methodological issues. For now, the most practical way to summarize the current evidence for medical cannabis for chronic pain is that a growing number of studies appear to support its use for certain types of pain but that a great deal of extrapolation must occur between medical literature and individual patients—since most studies are not evaluating the same products that are available to patients at cannabis dispensaries and retailers. In observational studies, patients with chronic, non-cancer pain who use medical cannabis report reduced opioid needs and improved QOL [13]. With appropriate dosing, cannabinoids may offer a more tolerable and safer analgesia compared to long-term opioids or non-steroidal anti-inflammatory medications.

4.4.2   Cancer Pain

Cannabis-based medicines may aid in the palliation of cancer-induced pain. Studies published over the past 15 years have examined multiple cannabis formulations, including oral THC, oral THC/CBD, oral CBD, and inhaled THC or whole-plant cannabis. Systematic reviews and meta-analyses of high-quality studies (i.e., RCTs) demonstrate conflicting results. For example, a 2020 meta-analysis indicated no difference in effectiveness compared to placebo when cannabinoids were added to opioids, while a 2017 systematic review and 2021 meta-analysis both concluded that the evidence showed dose-dependent analgesia from THC compared to placebo [14–16]. Published observational studies tend to be positive, showing improved analgesia and reduced use of opioid and non-opioid pain medications [17, 18]. Cannabis-based medicines continue to be of great interest as adjunct therapies for the palliation of advanced cancer pain.

4.4.3   Anxiety

Cannabis has long been utilized for the anecdotal management of anxiety symptoms. Preclinical studies have illustrated the role of the ECS in modulating mood and emotion. The pharmacologic response to exogenous cannabinoids activating CB_1 receptors is said to be "biphasic," with lower doses producing inhibitory and anxiolytic effects and higher doses producing anxiogenic effects and uncomfortable impairment from psychoactivity [19]. THC appears to be less helpful for anxiety symptoms for this reason. The non-impairing cannabinoid CBD appears to be both more effective and tolerable than THC for anxiety symptoms. Small studies have explored the effects of moderate doses of oral CBD given ahead of a stressful stimulus such as a medical test or public speaking. Participants reported reductions in anxiety, cognitive impairment, and physiologic discomfort [20]. Studies in which anxiety was evaluated as a secondary outcome also indicate that cannabinoids (both THC and CBD) may help improve anxiety associated with chronic pain [21].

4.4.4   Post-traumatic Stress Disorder (PTSD)

PTSD is a complex neurologic condition that causes psychological distress and functional impairment that persists following a traumatic event. Common symptoms include hypervigilance or heightened stress response, insomnia, mood dysregulation, and "flashbacks" [22]. Key roles of the ECS in PTSD are the modulation of stress responses, inhibition of emotional memories, and reduction of fear responses [23]. These features are well understood at the cellular level, but there is less clarity from clinical trials. Most larger studies are observational, and therefore, the results are less robust compared to RCTs. In some individual studies, veterans reported improvement and reduction in PTSD symptoms in response to different forms of cannabis, including synthetic nabilone, CBD, and whole-plant herbal cannabis [24–26]. However, a systematic review published in 2024 did not find major benefits, though cannabinoids may have a beneficial effect on some PTSD symptoms, such as flashbacks and reactivity. Additionally, the systematic review indicated that cannabinoids could be associated with a risk of serious negative effects, including worsening violent behavior or suicidal ideation [27]. Due to the large variety of formulations, doses, and responses and the lack of high-quality evidence, it is too early to confidently define the true efficacy and ideal dose and formulation of cannabis in the treatment of PTSD. Further research is needed to understand its therapeutic uses in this population.

4.4.5   Seizures and Spasticity

Seizures and spasticity are two common physiologic manifestations of neurologic and neurodegenerative conditions. A large body of research supports the efficacy of cannabinoids in the management of these symptoms. One of the most exciting developments in cannabis medicine in the last decade occurred when the FDA approved the first plant-derived cannabis product—CBD oil—for the treatment of the pediatric seizure disorders Dravet syndrome and Lennox-Gastaut syndrome [28]. Both are devastating genetic conditions with high mortality rates and shortened life expectancy. High-dose CBD in these patients seems to be well tolerated and effective in reducing seizure frequency and improving QOL. The most commonly reported side effects included somnolence and GI symptoms (nausea and diarrhea) [29]. There is also a significant risk of pharmacokinetic drug interactions with other anti-epileptic drugs, including clobazam and phenytoin, requiring close monitoring of symptoms and therapeutic drug levels [28].

Painful spasticity is another condition associated with numerous neurodegenerative conditions. The most well-studied of these in terms of the effects of cannabinoid medicine is multiple sclerosis (MS). Evaluations of cerebrospinal fluid of patients with MS indicate endocannabinoid deficiency and dysregulation [30]. A 2022 Cochrane review evaluated 25 RCTs, concluding that cannabinoids likely reduce the perceived severity of spasticity compared with placebo. Many of these studies were conducted in Europe and evaluated a pharmaceutical preparation of 1:1 THC/CBD oromucosal spray (nabiximols), with other studies evaluating synthetic THC (e.g., nabilone or dronabinol) or plant-based formulations [31]. Nabiximols is currently approved in several European countries and is in phase III trials in the US [32].

4.4.6   Appetite, Nausea, and Cachexia

Chronic and severe illnesses may impair appetite, food taste, GI motility, and nutrient absorption. The ECS plays an important role in regulating appetite control and the palatability and enjoyment of food [33]. Anecdotally, cannabis use has been associated with increased appetite ("munchies," anyone?). In the early 2000s, researchers sought to capitalize on this unintended effect of cannabinoid use by developing a CB_1 *antagonist* for use as a weight loss treatment. Rimonabant was successful as a weight loss drug and was approved in Europe, but trials were halted after serious neuropsychiatric adverse effects occurred, including one death by suicide. Rimonabant was never approved in the United States [34]. As for utilizing CB_1 *agonists* (i.e., THC) to increase food intake and promote weight gain in patients with severe diseases like cancer and human immunodeficiency virus (HIV)/acquired immunodeficiency syndrome (AIDS), results from RCTs are conflicting. Dronabinol (synthetic THC) demonstrated improved appetite, weight gain, and mood in clinical trials [35]. However, other investigations did not demonstrate symptom improvement with synthetic THC or were inferior to standard treatments like megestrol on weight gain and appetite [36, 37].

In the 1980s, studies found that a low-dose synthetic THC formulation reduced chemotherapy-induced nausea and vomiting effectively in multiple populations compared to placebo and was equivalent to the conventional antiemetic therapies at the time [38]. Subsequently, two preparations of synthetic THC, dronabinol and nabilone, were developed and have been on the market for this indication since the 1990s. They are both indicated for chemotherapy-induced nausea and vomiting, and dronabinol has an additional approved indication for anorexia associated with HIV/AIDS [39, 40].

4.4.7 Autism and Autism Spectrum Disorder (ASD)

ASD is a complex neurodevelopmental disorder that currently affects 3% of school-age children, though prevalence appears to be increasing [41]. There is currently intense interest and research exploring the role of the ECS in the development of ASD and the potential treatment of the disorder and its symptoms. Disturbances in cognition, mood, language, appetite, and sleep are prominent in children and adults with ASD [42]. Clinical studies of mixed methodologies have begun to explore the clinical efficacy of cannabinoids, primarily in mostly pediatric patients with ASD. Case series have suggested improvement in the core ASD symptoms described above with the use of CBD [43–45]. A 2023 randomized, double-blind, placebo-controlled trial of 60 ASD patients demonstrated significant improvement in social interaction, agitation, anxiety, and food intake in the treatment group that received CBD. Side effects included sedation, diarrhea, or paradoxical worsening of symptoms [46]. Current research with ongoing RCTs and larger sample sizes is essential to further understand the ideal role of cannabis-based medicines in the treatment of symptoms associated with ASD.

4.4.8 Quality of Life and Palliative Care

Due to the multisystem presence of CB receptors both centrally and peripherally, cannabinoids may have an important role in palliating symptoms commonly seen in advanced illness or near end-of-life. While we explored individual symptoms above, the holistic consideration of well-being and improved QOL remain vital endpoints in patient care, especially when no cure is available. End-of-life pain and symptoms also tend to be multifactorial, with added emotional and psychological stressors of loss of independence, dignity, and fear of dying. The palliative use of cannabis and cannabinoid-based medicines are of great clinical interest in this field. Commonly used pharmaceuticals for palliation at the end of life, including opioids, benzodiazepines, barbiturates, and antipsychotics, often come with intolerable side effects and the potential for overdose due to respiratory suppression.

Two systematic reviews published in 2018 and 2022, respectively, explored the effects of cannabis in palliative populations, with mixed findings. Cannabis was found to be inferior to megestrol in producing significant weight gain, with no significant improvement in caloric intake, findings which were considered low-quality evidence with a high risk of bias. Similar results were noted in the analysis of cannabinoid effects on nausea and vomiting, sleep, and cancer pain, with trends toward symptom reduction with cannabis use, but low-quality evidence and a high risk of bias [47]. The 2022 review evaluated cannabis' effect on QOL in various end-stage conditions, including 20 RCTs and 32 nonrandomized trials [48]. Positive treatment effects were reported in pain, nausea, appetite, sleep, fatigue, chemosensory perception, and night sweats but were considered low clinical significance and high risk of bias.

Although hospice patients overwhelmingly support the use of cannabis to treat end-of-life symptoms, hospice physicians approach this modality more cautiously. A national survey of hospice physicians in the United States in 2019 found that only half of the physicians ever certified patients for medical cannabis use and that many of those did so rarely (i.e., less than once per month) [49]. A 2023 survey of hospice and palliative medicine fellows found that although 83% received formal training in medical cannabis, only 20% felt confident in discussing cannabis or recommending cannabis use for patients [50].

4.5   But What About?

There are many other diagnoses for which cannabis is thought to help symptoms or with anecdotal reports and case reports of efficacy, but for which there is little or no evidence base on which to consider clinical use. A few of these are discussed below.

4.5.1   Glaucoma

One of the original conditions for which patients have reported improvement with cannabis use is glaucoma. That's because glaucoma patient and cannabis activist Robert Randall won a court case in 1975 allowing him to cultivate and use cannabis due to this medical necessity [51]. Since that time, many studies have attempted to prove the therapeutic value of cannabis to treat glaucoma, to no avail [52]. The American Academy of Ophthalmology recommends against self-treatment with cannabis or patients with glaucoma and does not endorse cannabis as an appropriate glaucoma treatment [53].

4.5.2 Depression

Depression is a common condition that often coexists with anxiety and other mental health conditions. While cannabis may reduce nervous system activation and the "fight or flight" response in these conditions, its role in improving depressive symptoms is unclear. In a few small studies, cannabis had no significant effect on depression in the setting of chronic pain or anxiety, and no currently published RCTs have evaluated cannabis treatment for depression as a primary outcome [54]. In fact, patients with coexisting conditions such as anxiety, bipolar disorder, or cannabis use disorder appear to be at higher risk for depression with cannabis use [55]. Despite the frequency with which patients seek out cannabis to treat depressive symptoms, further studies are needed to define the role of cannabis in depression.

4.5.3 Cancer

Another condition for which there is great interest in the role of cannabis in treatment is cancer. To date, the bulk of clinical evidence examines cannabis' effect on cancer-associated symptoms such as pain, anorexia, cachexia, and nausea/vomiting [7]. Studies evaluating cannabis extracts and cannabinoids as a primary or adjunctive treatment for cancer are still currently in the preclinical stage, with some promising in vitro findings but no clinical evidence to support recommending cannabis as a primary treatment for cancer.

> **Practice Tip: A Roadmap for Navigating Evidence-Based Medical Cannabis Care**
> - Step 1: Perform a complete history and physical exam, focusing on individual symptoms, characteristics, and treatment goals.
> - Step 2: Identify the key symptoms for which medical cannabis may be helpful.

- Step 3: Perform a literature search to identify the scope and strength of evidence for the desired condition:
  - *Research Tip*: Use multiple search term combinations to capture a wider range of studies. Example keywords: *cannabis*, *medical cannabis*, *cannabinoids*, *THC*, *CBD*, [and] the condition of interest.
  - *Research Tip*: Start with systematic reviews (i.e., the top of the evidence pyramid), which screen and capture the most relevant recent studies and often help discern methodologies and outcomes for interpretation.
  - *Research Tip*: Select high-quality RCTs mentioned in the review to see the details of patient characteristics, formulations, dosing, efficacy, and safety. Risk of bias is often high in cannabis studies, and cautious interpretation is needed.
- Step 4: Discern the strength of the evidence and decide on relevance to the current situation. If the patient is a good candidate and the condition may benefit from cannabinoid treatments, especially if multiple other treatments have failed, a trial of medical cannabis would be reasonable.
- Step 5: Using the expert consensus dosing recommendations, recommend the lowest initial dose ("start low and go slow"), with close monitoring and titration of response over the first 2–4 weeks. Encourage patients to use a symptom journal to track progress and effects. Chapter 8 of this book goes into greater detail about patient management.
- Step 6: Continue regular follow-up at least every 6 months, assessing cannabis use patterns, screening for adverse effects, monitoring for medication interactions, and overall effectiveness of medical cannabis products. Consider stopping medical cannabis treatment if no positive effects after multiple dose titrations or if intolerable side effects occur.

References

1. Levels of evidence. UC Davis Library Research Guides [Internet]. 2024. https://guides.library.ucdavis.edu/systematic-reviews/levels-of-evidence. Accessed 15 October 2024.
2. Suvarna V. Phase IV of drug development. Perspect Clin Res. 2010;1(2):57–60.
3. Azcarate PM, Zhang AJ, Keyhani S, Steigerwald S, Ishida JH, Cohen BE. Medical reasons for marijuana use, forms of use, and patient perception of physician attitudes among the US population. J Gen Intern Med. 2020;35(7):1979–86. https://doi.org/10.1007/s11606-020-05800-7.
4. Boehnke KF, Dean O, Haffajee RL, Hosanagar A. U.S. trends in registration for medical cannabis and reasons for use from 2016 to 2020: an observational study. Ann Intern Med. 2022;175(7):945–51. https://doi.org/10.7326/M22-0217.
5. Drug Enforcement Agency. Schedules of controlled substances: rescheduling of marijuana: a proposed rule by the Drug Enforcement Administration. 2024. https://www.federalregister.gov/documents/2024/05/21/2024-11137/schedules-of-controlled-substances-rescheduling-of-marijuana. Accessed 7 September 2024.
6. Sera L, Hempel-Sanderoff C. Cannabis science and therapeutics: an overview for clinicians. J Clin Pharmacol. 2024;64(5):499–513. https://doi.org/10.1002/jcph.2400.
7. National Academies of Sciences Engineering and Medicine. The health effects of cannabis and cannabinoids: the current state of evidence and recommendations for research. Washington: The National Academies Press; 2017. https://doi.org/10.17226/24625.
8. Hall A. CBD statistics, data and use (2023) – Forbes Health. 2023. https://www.forbes.com/health/body/cbd-statistics/. Accessed 7 September 2024.
9. Burston JJ, Woodhams SG. Endocannabinoid system and pain: an introduction. Proc Nutr Soc. 2014;73(1):106–17.
10. McDonagh MS, Morasco BJ, Wagner J, Ahmed AY, Fu R, Kansagara D, et al. Cannabis-based products for chronic pain: a systematic review. Ann Intern Med. 2022;175(8):1143–5.
11. Andreae MH, Carter GM, Shaparin N, Suslov K, Ellis RJ, Ware MA, et al. Inhaled cannabis for chronic neuropathic pain: a meta-analysis of individual patient data. J Pain. 2015;16(12):1221–32.
12. Linde LD, Ogryzlo CM, Choles CM, Cairns BE, Kramer JLK. Efficacy of topical cannabinoids in the management of pain: a systematic review and meta-analysis of animal studies. Reg Anesth Pain Med. 2022;47(3):183–91.
13. Noori A, Miroshnychenko A, Shergill Y, et al. Opioid-sparing effects of medical cannabis or cannabinoids for chronic pain: a systematic review

and meta-analysis of randomised and observational studies. BMJ Open. 2021;11:e047717. https://doi.org/10.1136/bmjopen-2020-047717.

14. Wang L, Hong PJ, May C, Rehman Y, Oparin Y, Hong CJ, Hong BY, AminiLari M, Gallo L, Kaushal A, Craigie S, Couban RJ, Kum E, Shanthanna H, Price I, Upadhye S, Ware MA, Campbell F, Buchbinder R, Agoritsas T, Busse JW. Medical cannabis or cannabinoids for chronic non-cancer and cancer related pain: a systematic review and meta-analysis of randomised clinical trials. BMJ. 2021;374:1034. https://doi.org/10.1136/bmj.n1034.

15. Tateo S. State of the evidence: cannabinoids and cancer pain—a systematic review. J Am Acad Nurse Pract. 2017;29(2):94–103.

16. Boland EG, Bennett MI, Allgar V, Boland JW. Cannabinoids for adult cancer-related pain: systematic review and meta-analysis. BMJ Support Palliat Care. 2020;10(1):14–24. https://doi.org/10.1136/bmjspcare-2019-002032. Epub 2020 Jan 20.

17. Cudmore J, Daeninck P. Use of medical cannabis to reduce pain and improve quality of life in cancer patients. J Clin Oncol. 2015;33(29):198. https://doi.org/10.1200/jco.2015.33.29_suppl.198.

18. Aviram J, Lewitus GM, Vysotski Y, Amna MA, Ouryvaev A, Procaccia S, et al. The effectiveness and safety of medical cannabis for treating cancer related symptoms in oncology patients. Front Pain Res. 2022;3:–861037.

19. Viveros MP, Marco EM, File SE. Endocannabinoid system and stress and anxiety responses. Pharmacol Biochem Behav. 2005;81(2):331–42. https://doi.org/10.1016/j.pbb.2005.01.029.

20. Stanciu CN, Brunette MF, Teja N, Budney AJ. Evidence for use of cannabinoids in mood disorders, anxiety disorders, and PTSD: a systematic review. Psychiatr Serv. 2021;72(4):429. https://doi.org/10.1176/APPI. PS.202000189.

21. Whiting PF, Wolff RF, Deshpande S, et al. Cannabinoids for medical use: a systematic review and meta-analysis. JAMA. 2015;313(24):2456–73. https://doi.org/10.1001/JAMA.2015.6358.

22. Orsolini L, Chiappini S, Volpe U, Berardis D, Latini R, Papanti GD, Corkery AJM. Use of medicinal cannabis and synthetic cannabinoids in post-traumatic stress disorder (PTSD): a systematic review. Medicina. 2019;55(9):525. https://doi.org/10.3390/medicina55090525. PMID: 31450833; PMCID: PMC6780141.

23. Jurkus R, Day HL, Guimarães FS, Lee JL, Bertoglio LJ, Stevenson CW. Cannabidiol regulation of learned fear: implications for treating anxiety-related disorders. Front Pharmacol. 2016;7:454. https://doi.org/10.3389/fphar.2016.00454. PMID: 27932983; PMCID: PMC5121237.

24. Earleywine M, Bolles JR. Marijuana, expectancies, and post-traumatic stress symptoms: a preliminary investigation. J Psychoactive Drugs. 2014;46(3):171–7. https://doi.org/10.1080/02791072.2014.920118.

25. Elms L, Shannon S, Hughes S, Lewis N. Cannabidiol in the treatment of post-traumatic stress disorder: a case series. J Altern Complement Med. 2019;25(4):392–7. https://doi.org/10.1089/acm.2018.0437. Epub 2018 Dec 13. PMID: 30543451; PMCID: PMC6482919.

26. Cameron C, Watson D, Robinson J. Use of a synthetic cannabinoid in a correctional population for posttraumatic stress disorder-related insomnia and nightmares, chronic pain, harm reduction, and other indications: a retrospective evaluation. J Clin Psychopharmacol. 2014;34(5):559–64. https://doi.org/10.1097/JCP.0000000000000180. PMID: 24987795; PMCID: PMC4165471.

27. Rodas JD, George TP, Hassan AN. A systematic review of the clinical effects of cannabis and cannabinoids in posttraumatic stress disorder symptoms and symptom clusters. J Clin Psychiatry. 2024;85(1):14862.

28. Sekar K, Pack A. Epidiolex as adjunct therapy for treatment of refractory epilepsy: a comprehensive review with a focus on adverse effects. F1000Res. 2019;8:234. https://doi.org/10.12688/f1000research.16515.1. PMID: 30854190; PMCID: PMC6396837.

29. Golub V, Reddy DS. Cannabidiol therapy for refractory epilepsy and seizure disorders. Adv Exp Med Biol. 2021;1264:93–110. https://doi.org/10.1007/978-3-030-57369-0_7.

30. Di Filippo M, Pini LA, Pelliccioli GP, Calabresi P, Sarchielli P. Abnormalities in the cerebrospinal fluid levels of endocannabinoids in multiple sclerosis. J Neurol Neurosurg Psychiatry. 2008;79(11):1224–9. https://doi.org/10.1136/jnnp.2007.139071. Epub 2008 Jun 5.

31. Filippini G, Minozzi S, Borrelli F, Cinquini M, Dwan K. Cannabis and cannabinoids for symptomatic treatment for people with multiple sclerosis. Cochrane Database Syst Rev. 2022;5(5):CD013444. https://doi.org/10.1002/14651858.CD013444.pub2. PMID: 35510826; PMCID: PMC9069991.

32. Meuth SG, Vila C, Dechant KL. Effect of Sativex on spasticity-associated symptoms in patients with multiple sclerosis. Expert Rev Neurother. 2015;15(8):909–18. https://doi.org/10.1586/14737175.2015.1067607. Epub 2015 Jul 11.

33. Jager G, Witkamp RF. The endocannabinoid system and appetite: relevance for food reward. Nutr Res Rev. 2014;27(1):172–85.

34. King A. Prevention: neuropsychiatric adverse effects signal the end of the line for rimonabant. Nat Rev Cardiol. 2010;7(11):602.

35. Beal JE, Olson R, Laubenstein L, Morales JO, Bellman P, Yangco B, et al. Dronabinol as a treatment for anorexia associated with weight loss in patients with AIDS. J Pain Symptom Manag. 1995;10(2):89–97.

36. Jatoi A, Windschitl HE, Loprinzi CL, Sloan JA, Dakhil SR, Mailliard JA, Pundaleeka S, Kardinal CG, Fitch TR, Krook JE, Novotny PJ, Christensen B. Dronabinol versus megestrol acetate versus combination therapy for cancer-associated anorexia: a North Central Cancer Treatment Group

study. J Clin Oncol. 2002;20(2):567–73. https://doi.org/10.1200/JCO.2002.20.2.567.

37. Timpone JG, Wright DJ, Li N, Egorin MJ, Enama ME, Mayers J, Galetto G. The safety and pharmacokinetics of single-agent and combination therapy with megestrol acetate and dronabinol for the treatment of HIV wasting syndrome. The DATRI 004 Study Group. Division of AIDS Treatment Research Initiative. AIDS Res Hum Retrovir. 1997;13(4):305–15. https://doi.org/10.1089/aid.1997.13.305.

38. May MB, Glode AE. Dronabinol for chemotherapy-induced nausea and vomiting unresponsive to antiemetics. Cancer Manag Res. 2016;8:49–55. https://doi.org/10.2147/CMAR.S81425. PMID: 27274310; PMCID: PMC4869612.

39. Dronabinol. Lexi-Drugs. UpToDate Lexidrug [Internet]. UpToDate Inc. https://online.lexi.com. Accessed 7 September 2024.

40. Nabilone. Lexi-drugs. UpToDate Lexidrug. UpToDate Inc. https://online.lexi.com. Accessed 7 September 2024.

41. Aran A, Cayam RD. Cannabinoid treatment for the symptoms of autism spectrum disorder. Expert Opin Emerg Drugs. 2024;29(1):65–79. https://doi.org/10.1080/14728214.2024.2306290. Epub 2024 Jan 23.

42. Maenner MJ, Warren Z, Williams AR, et al. Prevalence and characteristics of autism spectrum disorder among children aged 8 years—autism and developmental disabilities monitoring network, 11 sites, United States, 2020. MMWR Surveill Summ. 2023;72(2):1–14. https://doi.org/10.15585/mmwr.ss7202a1.

43. Hacohen M, Stolar OE, Berkovitch M, Elkana O, Kohn E, Hazan A, Heyman E, Sobol Y, Waissengreen D, Gal E, Dinstein I. Children and adolescents with ASD treated with CBD-rich cannabis exhibit significant improvements particularly in social symptoms: an open label study. Transl Psychiatry. 2022;12(1):375. https://doi.org/10.1038/s41398-022-02104-8. PMID: 36085294; PMCID: PMC9461457.

44. Fleury-Teixeira P, Caixeta FV, Ramires da Silva LC, Brasil-Neto JP, Malcher-Lopes R. Effects of CBD-enriched Cannabis sativa extract on autism spectrum disorder symptoms: an observational study of 18 participants undergoing compassionate use. Front Neurol. 2019;10:1145. https://doi.org/10.3389/fneur.2019.01145. PMID: 31736860; PMCID: PMC6834767.

45. Barchel D, Stolar O, De-Haan T, Ziv-Baran T, Saban N, Fuchs DO, Koren G, Berkovitch M. Oral cannabidiol use in children with autism spectrum disorder to treat related symptoms and co-morbidities. Front Pharmacol. 2019;9:1521. https://doi.org/10.3389/fphar.2018.01521. PMID: 30687090; PMCID: PMC6333745.

46. Montagner PSS, Medeiros W, da Silva LCR, Borges CN, Brasil-Neto J, de Deus Silva Barbosa V, Caixeta FV, Malcher-Lopes R. Individually tailored dosage regimen of full-spectrum Cannabis extracts for autistic core and comorbid symptoms: a real-life report of multi-symptomatic benefits.

Front Psych. 2023;14:1210155. https://doi.org/10.3389/fpsyt.2023.1210155. PMID: 37671290; PMCID: PMC10475955.

47. Mücke M, Weier M, Carter C, Copeland J, Degenhardt L, Cuhls H, Radbruch L, Häuser W, Conrad R. Systematic review and meta-analysis of cannabinoids in palliative medicine. J Cachexia Sarcopenia Muscle. 2018;9(2):220–34. https://doi.org/10.1002/jcsm.12273. Epub 2018 Feb 5. PMID: 29400010; PMCID: PMC5879974.

48. Doppen M, Kung S, Maijers I, John M, Dunphy H, Townsley H, Eathorne A, Semprini A, Braithwaite I. Cannabis in palliative care: a systematic review of current evidence. J Pain Symptom Manag. 2022;64(5):e260–84. https://doi.org/10.1016/j.jpainsymman.2022.06.002. Epub 2022 Jun 12.

49. Costantino RC, Felten N, Todd M, Maxwell T, McPherson ML. A survey of hospice professionals regarding medical cannabis practices. J Palliat Med. 2019;22(10):1208–12.

50. Sherry D, Patell R, Han HJ, Dodge LE, Braun I, Buss MK. Hospice and palliative medicine fellows' clinical discussions, perceived knowledge, and formal training regarding medical cannabis use: a national survey study (TH108B). J Pain Symptom Manag. 2023;65(3):e251–2.

51. Mack A, Joy J. Marijuana as medicine? The science beyond the controversy. Washington: National Academies Press; 2000. https://www.ncbi.nlm.nih.gov/books/NBK224398/. Accessed 7 September 2024.

52. National Eye Institute. Glaucoma and marijuana use [Internet]. 2005. https://www.nei.nih.gov/about/news-and-events/news/glaucoma-and-marijuana-use. Accessed 7 September 2024.

53. Tubert D, Gudgel D. Does marijuana help treat glaucoma and other eye conditions? [Internet] American Academy of Ophthalmology. 2023. https://www.aao.org/eye-health/tips-prevention/medical-marijuana-glaucoma-treament. Accessed 7 September 2024.

54. Sarris J, Sinclair J, Karamacoska D, Davidson M, Firth J. Medicinal cannabis for psychiatric disorders: a clinically-focused systematic review. BMC Psychiatry. 2020;20(1):24. https://doi.org/10.1186/s12888-019-2409-8. PMID: 31948424; PMCID: PMC6966847.

55. Petrilli K, Ofori S, Hines L, Taylor G, Adams S, Freeman TP. Association of cannabis potency with mental ill health and addiction: a systematic review. Lancet Psychiatry. 2022;9(9):736–50. https://doi.org/10.1016/S2215-0366(22)00161-4. Epub 2022 Jul 25.

Cannabis and Public Health: Safety Considerations in a Changing Landscape

5

5.1 Collecting and Evaluating Public Health Data

One undeniable truth about integrating cannabis into modern Western medical practice is that policies enabling broader access to cannabis products have been developed even though we lack a full understanding of the benefits and risks of cannabis use. That's not typically how we do things in the US, where the FDA approves products only after pharmaceutical companies provide "substantial evidence of effectiveness" from research that includes one "adequate and well-controlled clinical trial" [1]. What effect have these policies had on public health? What concerns must be addressed as restrictions loosen and access increases? This chapter discusses public health issues, including cannabis use disorder, impaired driving drug testing, maternal cannabis use, emergency room visits, and hospitalizations related to cannabis adverse effects, adolescent non-medical use and pediatric exposures, and quality control of cannabis products.

Data on public health issues is typically collected via observational research. Types of observational studies include cohort, cross-sectional, and case-control studies. In a cohort study, two groups of participants, one group with a certain exposure (say, tobacco use) and one group without the exposure (no tobacco use), are followed for a period of time (say, 10 years). The fre-

© The Author(s), under exclusive license to Springer Nature Switzerland AG 2025
L. Sera, C. Hempel-Sanderoff, *Cannabis Science and Therapeutics*, https://doi.org/10.1007/978-3-031-80352-9_5

quency with which the exposed group experiences a predefined outcome (say, lung cancer) is compared to the frequency of the outcome in the unexposed group. In this study, the investigators aren't introducing any treatment or controlling the groups in any way—they are simply observing the outcome. In a case-control study, investigators look backward in time in a population of patients with or without the outcome of interest (lung cancer) to determine the relative frequencies of exposure in both groups. These are both very different from experimental studies (e.g., RCTs), where a group of participants are randomized into either the experimental group (receives an investigational treatment) or a control group (receives a placebo). The treatment setting is tightly controlled in an experimental study, and the participant population is carefully chosen.

There are many benefits of observational studies. Such studies are less expensive than RCTs, are more efficient for studying rare diseases, and are sometimes the only ethical way to study certain conditions, especially harms. The study population is often more reflective of the real world (i.e., more generalizable). The downside is that observational studies are much more prone to bias (systematic errors in methodology that distort the accuracy of the study results) than RCTs. RCTs have high internal validity (low risk of bias) but low external validity (less generalizable to a real-world population). One of the main concerns with observational studies is confounding. A confounding variable confuses our conclusions about the association between the exposure and the outcome of interest. For instance, let's say I wanted to study the association between smoking cannabis and developing lung cancer. I take a group of individuals who smoke cannabis and a group of individuals who don't smoke cannabis, follow them for 10 years, and see how many in each group have developed lung cancer. Sounds simple, right? But what if the people who smoke cannabis are also more likely to smoke tobacco than the group who doesn't smoke cannabis? We know that tobacco smoke is a risk factor for lung cancer. That means that even if we find that individuals who smoke cannabis are more likely to develop lung cancer, we can't be sure how much of that effect is truly due to tobacco smoke unless we control for the confounding variable, either in our participant selection or by statistical analysis. Due to the presence of potential confounders, we can never say with confidence that there is a *causal relationship* between an exposure and an outcome in an observational study. If we knew with certainty that we had identified and controlled for every possible confounder, we could determine causality—but we can't. Therefore, the best we can say is that there is or is not an *association* between an exposure and a confounder.

Most studies exploring cannabis harms and public health are observational studies. Therefore, we can determine the presence of associations between cannabis use and certain outcomes, but generally not causality. Additionally, most studies exploring harms and public health concerns related to cannabis either target populations who use cannabis for non-medical (i.e., recreational purposes) or make no distinction between those who use cannabis for medical purposes and those who do not. Additionally, defining what constitutes "medical" and "non-medical" use is challenging. Sometimes, participants say that they use cannabis for both medical and non-medical reasons [2]. The bottom line is that we need to be very clear about how we interpret the cannabis scientific literature with regard to the effects of using cannabis medically.

5.2   Cannabis Use Disorder

Cannabis use disorder (CUD), like any substance use disorder, is characterized by compulsive cannabis use that continues despite harmful consequences. According to the *Diagnostic and Statistical Manual of Mental Disorders* (DSM-5), patients can be diagnosed with CUD if they experienced at least two of the indicators in Table 5.1 within a 12-month period [3]. The DSM-5 criteria are broad and encompass a range of severity from mild to moderate impairment. The rate of CUD among participants who use cannabis for medical purposes is about 25%, according to a meta-analysis published in 2024 that evaluated 14 published studies, most of which relied on self-report to identify problematic cannabis use. Younger patients (under age 30) and individuals who use medical cannabis and also have chronic pain, mood disorders, PTSD, or psychotic disorder may be at higher risk for developing CUD [4]. The most frequently reported indicators of

Table 5.1 Indicators of cannabis use disorder [3]

Using larger amounts of cannabis than intended or using for longer duration than intended
History of unsuccessful attempts to reduce or quit cannabis use
Spending excessive time acquiring and using cannabis or recovering from cannabis effects
Experiencing cannabis cravings
Compulsive use and neglect of social obligations
Skipping social, occupational, or recreational activities to use cannabis
Continued use despite adverse social consequences
Continued use despite adverse physical consequences
Tolerance to the effects of cannabis (typically leading to larger amounts used)
Experiencing withdrawal symptoms during periods of abstinence

CUD are cannabis tolerance (the need for increased consumption to achieve the desired effect) and withdrawal (the experience of physical and psychiatric symptoms associated with abrupt cessation after prolonged cannabis use) [3, 4]. Although rates of cannabis use and CUD among adults increased in states where medical or recreational cannabis was legal, the prevalence of teen cannabis use has remained stable [5–7]. CUD is discussed further in Sect. 7.4.

5.3   Impaired Driving and Accidents in the Workplace

One of the foremost public health concerns in states that have legalized cannabis use (especially for non-medical use) is whether enacting such laws leads to a related increase in traffic fatalities. The psychoactive effects of THC, such as impaired motor coordination, attention, and concentration and slower decision-making ability, may increase the risk of accidents and injuries. Studies investigating the effect of cannabinoids on driving indicate that THC-containing cannabis products lead to impaired driving. Products with a higher concentration of CBD compared to THC (i.e., CBD-dominant formulations) did not significantly impact driving ability compared to placebo, but products with equal amounts of THC and CBD were as intoxicating as THC alone—the presence of CBD did not attenuate the psychoactive effects of THC [8, 9]. Both inhaled and edible THC-containing products can produce intoxication that may impair driving ability—and edible formulations have a slower onset of action and longer duration of action compared to smoked or vaporized cannabis products [10]. The literature is mixed regarding the impact of cannabis legalization on traffic fatalities, possibly because there is no standard definition of cannabis-related impairment or standardized testing methodology for impairment [6]. Similarly, studies evaluating the effect of cannabis use on workplace accidents and injuries have conflicting results [11]. A recent study of Canadian workers indicates that cannabis use increased the risk of injury only when the cannabis was used while an individual was *at work*—respondents who used cannabis outside the workplace had no higher risk of injuries than respondents with no past-year use [12].

5.3.1   And What about Drug Testing?

The pharmacokinetic and pharmacodynamic profiles of cannabis make it challenging for employers or law enforcement officials to differentiate cannabis impairment from cannabis exposure. Unlike blood alcohol levels, which are associated with typical physiological and cognitive effects, there is no such standard measurement to quantify or qualify cannabis impairment. This is certainly not due to a lack of trying; studies have evaluated dozens of roadside screening assessments, including oral fluid, urine, and behavioral tests [13]. Because the half-life of THC is 1 day in infrequent cannabis users and 5–10 days in frequent cannabis users, individuals may test positive for THC and its metabolites even when not acutely impaired. Furthermore, studies show a very weak, weak, or moderate association between blood/oral fluid concentration of THC/THC metabolites and subjective reports of impairment in occasional cannabis users and no significant association in regular users [14]. So far, no reliable testing method has been found to identify acute impairment.

> **Practice Tip**
> Remind patients that even if they are certified and registered participants in a state's legal medical cannabis program, employers can still enforce workplace bans on cannabis. Few states have legal protections for workers who are legally using medical cannabis. Patients should be aware of state laws, protections (where available), and workplace policies.

5.4   Use During Pregnancy and Breastfeeding

As cannabis use becomes more acceptable in society, the perception that it is "natural and therefore safe" may lead to increased use among pregnant and breastfeeding women. As of 2019, about 5% of pregnant women in the United Sates use cannabis, according to the Substance Abuse and Mental Health Services Administration [15]. Women who use cannabis during pregnancy report doing so primarily for management of pregnancy-related symptoms such as nausea and vomiting, even if they used cannabis before pregnancy for other reasons (i.e., enjoyment and/or management of life stressors) [16]. Cannabinoids are accepted as an effective treatment for chemotherapy-induced nausea and vomiting, and pregnant women may also turn to cannabis to alleviate pregnancy-related nausea and vomiting. About 14% of women with hyperemesis gravidarum, a syndrome of intractable vomiting during pregnancy, reported using cannabis for relief in a 2021 survey [17]. Pregnant women may also use cannabis to manage stress, anxiety, or pain [18].

THC readily crosses the placenta, with fetal plasma concentrations about 10% of maternal concentrations. Fetal concentrations may be higher with regular maternal use [19]. The body of evidence evaluating the harms of cannabis use during pregnancy is challenging to interpret. Because it would be unethical to conduct an RCT involving pregnant women and cannabis, all the available data comes from observational studies. While observational (cohort, cross-sectional, and case-control) studies have their place in evidence-based medicine, they are prone to bias and confounding. For instance, most studies rely on self-report of cannabis use, a methodology that may lead to underestimation. There are many potential confounders (education and income level and exposure to other drugs, alcohol, and tobacco, to name a few) in such studies that may cloud the associations between cannabis use and reported outcomes. As in other observational studies, there is little distinction between medical and non-medical cannabis use.

With that in mind, the published data indicate several potential short- and long-term harms associated with using cannabis during pregnancy. Cannabis use during pregnancy has been associated with low birth weight and adverse neurodevelopmental outcomes [20]. Cannabis smoke contains the same toxic compounds as tobacco smoke, and the available evidence doesn't enable comparisons in risk between inhaled and oral cannabis formulations. Cannabinoids and metabolites (THC, 11-OH-THC, 11-COOH-THC, CBD, and CBN) can be detected in breast milk. Due to the potential for harm and the lack of data with which to draw conclusions about the effects of cannabis during pregnancy and lactation, the American College of Obstetricians and Gynecologists discourages cannabis use. Cannabis use during pregnancy is also discussed in Sect. 7.4.

Practice Tip
Talk to pregnant patients using respectful, non-judgmental language. While women may be more open to discussing cannabis use, given the shift toward public acceptance, stigma remains. Concerns about reporting requirements to child protective services or data registries may prevent some women from candidly discussing cannabis use. If a patient is unable or unwilling to stop, advise reducing the frequency of use while pregnant and breastfeeding.

5.5   Adolescent Non-medical Use

Reducing non-medical cannabis use among teens is a major public health concern. The rapidly growing public acceptance of cannabis medical and non-medical use, coupled with increasing access to cannabis products, may give teens the erroneous impression that cannabis is completely safe. However, cannabis use is associated with some risks specific to adolescents and their growing brains. Remember from Chap. 1 that the ECS is intricately involved in the homeostasis of the nervous system. CB receptors are present in many brain structures and are highly concentrated in the frontal and limbic lobes (involved in executive function, learning, memory, and emotion) [21]. The teen years are a critical time for brain development, especially of the prefrontal cortex, and development may continue into the early 20 s. This is not a good time for teens to be messing around with their endocannabinoid systems by altering them with phytocannabinoids.

Heavy cannabis use during the teen years may alter the physical structure of brain matter as well as brain function. Exposure to cannabis may be associated with short-term and long-term neurocognitive effects. However, as with many studies of cannabis-related harms, the relationships between cannabis use and cognitive function are clouded by confounding, and most studies have evaluated the effects of non-medical use of cannabis (or haven't differentiated between medical and non-medical use). Additionally, cannabis is more potent (i.e., has a higher concentration of THC) now than it used to be—and we don't know how that might influence any of these cognitive outcomes. Pediatric use of medical cannabis is addressed in Sect. 7.4.

Practice Tip
Discourage non-medical cannabis use in individuals under age 25. Talk candidly with patients (and parents if appropriate) about the risks versus benefits of using cannabis if medically indicated—including transparency about the lack of conclusive evidence related to adolescent cannabis use and neurocognitive effects. Use CBD-only products if possible.

5.6   Quality Control, Packaging, and Labeling

Quality control of cannabis products through analytical testing is critical to ensure their safety. Cannabis products are medications. As such, healthcare providers and patients need to know what is in the products they recommend and use, and the products must be clearly and accurately labeled. Analytical testing of cannabis products encompasses the determination of the presence and potency of different cannabinoids and terpenes and the quantifying of heavy metals, pesticides, microorganisms (bacteria, yeast, mold), and other contaminants. Cannabis products may be contaminated at several points in their life cycle: cultivators use pesticides to protect plants from pathogens; processors use chemical solvents to make extracts; plants may contain bacteria, mold, and other microbiological impurities. Determining acceptable limits of impurities requires a lot of back and forth between regulators and cultivators. When acceptable levels are set too low, few or none of the tested products pass. This, in turn, leads to bad actors attempting to cheat the system (and at least sometimes succeeding) by "lab shopping" (sending products to multiple labs and using the passing results) or by sending irradiated samples to be tested (since radiation kills all the microorganisms).

Currently, each state with a legal cannabis program develops policies and regulations regarding quality control, including which contaminants to test for and acceptable levels of different contaminants. Most, but not all, states require some type of analytical testing of cannabis products sold in the state market. However, there is currently no universal standard to guide the development of testing programs (though the US Pharmacopeia is in the process of reincarnating the cannabis monograph for the first time since it was removed from the compendium in 1942—see Chap. 6 for a discussion of cannabis regulatory history in the United States).

As with testing limits and processes, no standard exists for packaging and labeling of cannabis products; states develop their own guidance and policies. The standard dose or serving size varies between states, generally 5 or 10 mg THC. However, cannabis products—particularly edible products—may contain 10 or 20 such doses. Labels may be unclear or require the user to have numeracy (the ability to work with numbers) to determine the appropriate dose. This could lead to dosing misadventures. The rate of cannabis exposures reported to the US National Poison Data System (for instance, when the Poison Center gets a call about an adult who ate a chocolate bar containing 100 mg of THC because they didn't know the dose was one-tenth of the bar or a kindergartener polished off a container full of colorful gummy candies that each contained 5 mg THC) increased by 67–77% once states opened a legal cannabis market [22].

> **Practice Tip**
> As a harm reduction measure, advise patients using canna-
> bis products to use only those products at a legal commer-
> cial establishment. Though testing and labeling requirements
> could (and should) be improved, these products are safer
> than unregulated products sold on the black market—and
> those sold on the gray market (for instance, the hemp-
> derived delta-8-THC products sold in gas stations and
> smoke shops).

References

1. US Food and Drug Administration. FDA issues draft guidance regarding confirmatory evidence of clinical trials [internet]. 2023. Accessed 28 Aug 2024.   https://www.fda.gov/drugs/drug-safety-and-availability/fda-issues-draft-guidance-regarding-confirmatory-evidence-clinical-trials.
2. Lin LA, Ilgen MA, Jannausch M, Bohnert KM. Comparing adults who use cannabis medically with those who use recreationally: results from a national sample. Addict Behav. 2016;61:99–103. https://doi.org/10.1016/j.addbeh.2016.05.015. Epub 2016 May 17. PMID: 27262964; PMCID: PMC4915997.
3. Patel J, Marwaha R. Cannabis use disorder. In: StatPearls. Treasure Island, FL: StatPearls Publishing; 2022. https://www.ncbi.nlm.nih.gov/books/NBK538131/.
4. Dawson D, Stjepanović D, Lorenzetti V, Cheung C, Hall W, Leung J. The prevalence of cannabis use disorders in people who use medicinal cannabis: a systematic review and meta-analysis. Drug Alcohol Depend. 2024;257:111263.   https://doi.org/10.1016/j.drugalcdep.2024.111263. Epub 2024 Mar 8.
5. Bailey JA, Tiberio SS, Kerr DCR, Epstein M, Henry KL, Capaldi DM. Effects of cannabis legalization on adolescent cannabis use across 3 studies. Am J Prev Med. 2023;64(3):361–7. https://doi.org/10.1016/j.amepre.2022.09.019. Epub 2022 Nov 10. PMID: 36372654; PMCID: PMC9975019.
6. Chiu V, Leung J, Hall W, Stjepanović D, Degenhardt L. Public health impacts to date of the legalisation of medical and recreational cannabis use in the USA. Neuropharmacology. 2021;193:108610. https://doi.org/10.1016/j.neuropharm.2021.108610.

7. Hall W, Stjepanović D, Caulkins J, et al. Public health implications of legalising the production and sale of cannabis for medicinal and recreational use. Lancet. 2019;394(10208):1580–90. https://doi.org/10.1016/S0140-6736(19)31789-1.

8. Arkell TR, Lintzeris N, Kevin RC, Ramaekers JG, Vandrey R, Irwin C, Haber PS, McGregor IS. Cannabidiol (CBD) content in vaporized cannabis does not prevent tetrahydrocannabinol (THC)-induced impairment of driving and cognition. Psychopharmacology (Berl). 2019;236(9):2713–24. https://doi.org/10.1007/s00213-019-05246-8. Epub 2019 May 1. PMID: 31044290; PMCID: PMC6695367.

9. Arkell TR, Vinckenbosch F, Kevin RC, Theunissen EL, McGregor IS, Ramaekers JG. Effect of cannabidiol and Δ9-tetrahydrocannabinol on driving performance: a randomized clinical trial. JAMA. 2020;324(21):2177–86. https://doi.org/10.1001/jama.2020.21218.

10. Zhao S, Brands B, Kaduri P, Wickens CM, Hasan OSM, Chen S, Le Foll B, Di Ciano P. The effect of cannabis edibles on driving and blood THC. J Cannabis Res. 2024;6(1):26. https://doi.org/10.1186/s42238-024-00234-y. PMID: 38822413; PMCID: PMC11140993.

11. Biasutti WR, Leffers KSH, Callaghan RC. Systematic review of cannabis use and risk of occupational injury. Subst Use Misuse. 2020;55(11):1733–45. https://doi.org/10.1080/10826084.2020.1759643. Epub 2020 May 22.

12. Carnide N, Landsman V, Lee H, Frone MR, Furlan AD, Smith PM. Workplace and non-workplace cannabis use and the risk of workplace injury: findings from a longitudinal study of Canadian workers. Can J Public Health. 2023;114(6):947–55.

13. Wennberg E, Windle SB, Filion KB, Thombs BD, Gore G, Benedetti A, Grad R, Ells C, Eisenberg MJ. Roadside screening tests for cannabis use: a systematic review. Heliyon. 2023;9(4):e14630. https://doi.org/10.1016/j.heliyon.2023.e14630. PMID: 37064483; PMCID: PMC10102219.

14. McCartney D, Arkell TR, Irwin C, Kevin RC, McGregor IS. Are blood and oral fluid Δ9-tetrahydrocannabinol (THC) and metabolite concentrations related to impairment? A meta-regression analysis. Neurosci Biobehav Rev. 2022;134:104433.

15. Substance Abuse and Mental Health Services Administration. Key substance use and mental health indicators in the United States: results from the 2019 National Survey on Drug Use and Health (HHS Publication No. PEP20-07-01-001, NSDUH Series H-55) [Internet]. Rockville, MD: Center for Behavioral Health Statistics and Quality, Substance Abuse and Mental Health Services Administration; 2020. https://www.samhsa.gov/data/.

16. Vanstone M, Taneja S, Popoola A, Panday J, Greyson D, Lennox R, McDonald SD. Reasons for cannabis use during pregnancy and lactation: a qualitative study. CMAJ. 2021;193(50):E1906–14. https://doi.org/10.1503/cmaj.211236. Erratum in: CMAJ 2022 Mar 7;194(9):E342. doi: 10.1503/cmaj.220230. PMID: 34930765; PMCID: PMC8687504.

17. First OK, MacGibbon KW, Cahill CM, Cooper ZD, Gelberg L, Cortessis VK, Mullin PM, Fejzo MS. Patterns of use and self-reported effectiveness of cannabis for hyperemesis gravidarum. Geburtshilfe Frauenheilkd. 2022;82(5):517–27. https://doi.org/10.1055/a-1749-5391. PMID: 35528189; PMCID: PMC9076215.
18. Ko JY, Coy KC, Haight SC, Haegerich TM, Williams L, Cox S, Njai R, Grant AM. Characteristics of marijuana use during pregnancy—eight states, pregnancy risk assessment monitoring system, 2017. MMWR Morb Mortal Wkly Rep. 2020;69(32):1058–63. https://doi.org/10.15585/mmwr.mm6932a2. PMID: 32790656; PMCID: PMC7440118.
19. Hutchings DE, Martin BR, Gamagaris Z, Miller N, Fico T. Plasma concentrations of delta-9-tetrahydrocannabinol in dams and fetuses following acute or multiple prenatal dosing in rats. Life Sci. 1989;44(11):697–701. https://doi.org/10.1016/0024-3205(89)90380-9.
20. Committee Opinion No. 722. American College of Obstetricians and Gynecologists. Marijuana use during pregnancy and lactation. Obstet Gynecol. 2017;130:e205–9.
21. Glass M, Faull RLM, Dragunow M. Cannabinoid receptors in the human brain: a detailed anatomical and quantitative autoradiographic study in the fetal, neonatal and adult human brain. Neuroscience. 1997;77(2):299–318.
22. Shi Y, Liang D. The association between recreational cannabis commercialization and cannabis exposures reported to the US National Poison Data System. Addiction. 2020;115(10):1890–9. https://doi.org/10.1111/add.15019. Epub 2020 Mar 10. PMID: 32080937; PMCID: PMC7438241.

Cannabis Regulations in the United States: A (Very) Brief Overview

6

6.1   Past Is Prologue

In August 2023, something happened in Washington, DC, that sent shockwaves through anyone paying attention to the cannabis regulatory landscape. The Department of Health and Human Services (HHS) representative sent a letter to the Drug Enforcement Administration (DEA) recommending that cannabis be removed from Schedule I under the CSA and reclassified as a Schedule III drug under the Act [1]. The CSA defines Schedule I substances as those that have the highest potential for addiction and no accepted medical use. In contrast, Schedule III drugs have an accepted medical use and lower potential for physical and psychological dependence [2]. In May 2024, the DEA agreed to move forward with rescheduling, a move that acknowledges decades of scientific advancement and has implications for research and medicine. But how did we get here? This chapter provides an overview of cannabis regulatory history in the United States along with perspectives on the future of cannabis policy.

Cannabis has a long history as a plant used in both medicine and industry. As we touched on in Chap. 2, historical artifacts dating back thousands of years describe how cannabis preparations were used for conditions such as pain, mood, and fatigue in many ancient cultures [3]. Cannabis became a popular remedy in Europe in the nineteenth century during the British colonization of India, and

75

L. Sera, C. Hempel-Sanderoff, *Cannabis Science and Therapeutics*, https://doi.org/10.1007/978-3-031-80352-9_6

European physicians studied its effects as an analgesic, anticonvulsant, and antiemetic [3]. In 1850, cannabis was added to the US Pharmacopeia (USP), a compilation of strength, purity, quality, and consistency standards for drugs, dietary supplements, and food ingredients [4]. Because cannabis was included in the USP, it was legal and regulated under the Pure Food and Drug Act of 1906 [5].

In the early decades of the twentieth century, the US government regulated narcotics such as cocaine and opium through taxation and, increasingly, criminal penalties [6]. In 1930, Harry Anslinger was named commissioner of the Bureau of Narcotics, a forerunner of the DEA, and this appointment had a profound effect on the regulation of cannabis in the United States into the 1960s. Anslinger exploited racial tensions resulting from large-scale immigration from Mexico after the Mexican-American War of the 1840s to consolidate support for anti-cannabis legislation [6]. The Marihuana Tax Act of 1937 essentially prohibited the use of cannabis as a medical treatment due to hefty taxes on medical use and heftier fines for violations of the Act [6]. Cannabis was removed from the USP in 1942. Although some policymakers and physicians challenged the idea that cannabis was a dangerous drug with no medical value, most notably in the La Guardia Report of 1944, US drug policy advanced toward increasingly severe criminal penalties for drug use [7].

6.1.1   The Controlled Substances Act and Modern Cannabis Regulation

In 1961, the Single Convention on Narcotic Drugs set international regulations and standards for drugs, including placing cannabis in Schedule I, denoting it as highly addictive and under the strictest controls [8]. Passed in 1970, the CSA created drug schedules under US law that mirrored the Single Convention [7]. Congress sorted drugs into five schedules under the CSA, placing cannabis in Schedule I, where it has remained to the present day (as of this writing). Drugs classified as Schedule I may not be prescribed, dispensed, or administered in the course of clinical practice [9]. Researchers intending to investigate the clinical potential of Schedule I substances face regulatory, funding, and supply challenges.

Table 6.1 Petitions to reschedule cannabis [10, 11]

Year submitted	Petitioners	Year denied
1972	National Organization for the reform of marijuana Laws (NORML)	1989
1995	Jon Gettman (director of NORML) and *high times* magazine	2001
2002	Coalition for Rescheduling Cannabis	2011
2011	Governors of Rhode Island and Washington	2016

That cannabis remained a Schedule I substance for so long despite steadily increasing public acceptance of its medical value is not due to a lack of effort on the part of advocacy groups and individuals. Since 1970, four petitions have been filed with the DEA requesting cannabis be removed from Schedule I (Table 6.1) [10, 11]. The first of these, filed in 1972 by the National Organization for the Reform of Marijuana Laws (NORML), went through years of litigation before finally being denied by the DEA in 1989 [10]. In the face of federal inaction, many jurisdictions have pursued policy change at the state level. California was the first state to legalize cannabis for medical use through a ballot measure called the Compassionate Use Act in 1996 [11]. Since then, other states have followed suit, and as of 2024, 38 states, 3 territories, and Washington, DC, permit the medical use of cannabis [12].

The disconnect between federal and state cannabis laws resulted, perhaps surprisingly, given the vehement criminalization of cannabis in the twentieth century, in the US government more or less turning a blind eye to state cannabis reform in the twenty-first. At first, the Department of Justice (DOJ) tried to enforce the CSA for early adopters of medical cannabis legalization, such as California, Washington, Oregon, and Colorado, shutting down cannabis farms and dispensaries. However, this approach ultimately floundered, largely due to the rapid advancement of public support for cannabis legalization and the fact that shuttered operations were quickly replaced [13]. In 2009, the DOJ issued guidance to US attorneys that federal resources should not be used to prosecute "individuals whose actions are in clear and unambiguous compliance with existing state laws providing for the medical use of marijuana" [14]. The Rohrabacher-Farr amendment, which blocked the DOJ from using funds to "prevent [states, territories, and Washington, DC] from implementing their own laws" related to the cultivation, distribution, and possession of cannabis, was signed into law in 2014 [15]. Though there have been many other congressional attempts to pass federal medical cannabis reform (starting in 1981), none has so far succeeded in moving cannabis from Schedule I [6].

6.2   So What Happens When Cannabis Is Rescheduled?

Rescheduling cannabis would be the most impactful change in federal cannabis regulation in nearly a hundred years and has implications for research, medical practice, and product regulation—but what might that look like?

6.2.1   Fewer Hurdles to Conducting Research

The research process for Schedule I drugs is administratively challenging, time-consuming, and complex. All investigators researching controlled substances must register with the DEA, in addition to obtaining a state license and institutional permission to conduct such research [16]. Researchers who wish to work with Schedule I drugs must submit all research protocols to the DEA for approval, and changes to the protocol must also be submitted and approved. In the United States, there are a limited number of cultivation facilities supplying cannabis for research purposes; the DEA takes possession of all cannabis crops and is responsible for distributing all such cannabis to investigators [17]. Grant funding is hard to obtain, and many publicly funded universities and laboratories do not support research with Schedule I drugs [18]. Moving cannabis to Schedule III would remove many administrative hurdles to conducting research. What rescheduling *doesn't* do—and this is important—is automatically classify every existing cannabis product (even those legally sold in state markets) as a Schedule III substance. It's still going to be a challenge to conduct research on the products that most patients can purchase and use from the state market.

6.2.2   A Cultural Shift in Medical Practice

A less tangible but no less important impact would be a cultural shift in how cannabis is perceived by the medical community. We really, really hope this happens. By rescheduling cannabis, the US government is acknowledging that cannabis has accepted medical uses and should be regulated as a therapeutic entity. Most healthcare providers are unprepared to answer questions about cannabis or counsel patients on its use, and those who don't support cannabis-based medicine often cite a lack of medical evidence as a reason [19]. Rescheduling may alleviate ethical and legal concerns of the medical community, increasing physicians' comfort in discussing cannabis with patients and their interest in learning about the plant and its therapeutic properties. Even when cannabis was a Schedule I drug, physicians were allowed to discuss cannabis with patients and recommend it as a medical therapy in states where use is legal. However, without a legal prescription, cannabis retailers don't have to dispense a specific product, regardless of what is recommended by the physician. Additionally, medical cannabis products aren't considered covered expenses by commercial insurance policies, Medicare, or Medicaid. The cost of cannabis products is a major concern for patients, and many states require patients to obtain certification from a healthcare provider and register with the state regulatory agency—expenses that also are not covered by insurance [20].

To be clear, rescheduling cannabis doesn't make it legal for physicians (or other prescribers) to write prescriptions for the non-FDA-approved cannabis products currently being sold in dispensaries, nor would it make the purchase of such products by individuals for medical or non-medical use legal under federal law. Under existing regulations, physicians would still only be able to write prescriptions for FDA-approved products. Currently, there are three FDA-approved cannabinoid products on the market: plant-derived CBD and the synthetic THC products dronabinol and nabilone. Dronabinol is a Schedule III substance and nabilone is a Schedule II substance. When CBD oil was approved in June 2018, CBD was a Schedule I substance (because it was derived from cannabis, which is a Schedule I substance). In September 2018, the DEA rescheduled CBD oil, placing it on Schedule V (the least restrictive schedule) [21]. In 2020, the DEA descheduled CBD oil, and it is now regulated like any other non-controlled prescription drug [22]. All other forms of CBD, except for those derived from hemp, remain restricted under the CSA [23]. Under the less complex and challenging requirements for researching Schedule III substances, pharmaceutical companies might be more likely to invest the time and expense in developing new cannabinoid prescription drugs, which would then be eligible for coverage under insurance policies—but this remains to be seen. There are currently no FDA-approved full-spectrum botanical products on the market.

6.2.3   Tax Equity for Cannabis Businesses

Congress created the Internal Revenue Service Section 280E in the 1980s after a convicted drug trafficker won a court case that allowed the illegal business to deduct expenses such as rent and packaging materials [24]. Section 280E prohibits businesses from deducting expenses or claiming tax credits from selling Schedule I or Schedule II substances [25]. This means that cannabis businesses, though operating legally in the state market, must pay federal taxes based on their gross income rather than taxable income after deducting business expenses. With cannabis as a Schedule III substance, businesses will be able to deduct expenses and enjoy a much lower tax liability.

6.3   Why Is Rescheduling Happening Now?

Given the long history of inaction by the federal government regarding rescheduling, the 2023 recommendation to reschedule came as a surprise. However, it was presumably related to

Table 6.2   Elements that constitute "currently accepted medical use" [27]

Element	Acceptable evidence
Drug's chemistry is known and reproducible	Substance is listed in an official compendium
Drug is safe	Adequate safety studies
Drug is effective	Adequate, well-controlled studies proving efficacy
The drug is accepted by qualified experts	Substance has an NDA approved by the FDA
Scientific evidence is widely available	In the absence of an NDA, evidence of safety and efficacy is widely available in sufficient detail

President Biden's October 2022 directive to HHS to "initiate the administrative process to review expeditiously how marijuana is classified under federal law" [26].

Before 2023, the last HHS scientific review of cannabis was conducted in response to the most recent petition to reschedule cannabis, submitted by the governors of Rhode Island and Washington in 2011. At that time, HHS concluded in 2015 that cannabis should not be rescheduled because it met the definition of a Schedule I drug based on a scientific evaluation of five elements that characterize a "currently accepted medical treatment" (CAMU) (Table 6.2) [28]. In its letter to the DEA, HHS conceded that cannabis research had progressed between 2006 (the year of the preceding evaluation) and 2015 and that this research generated a substantial body of evidence for the therapeutic applications of cannabis. However, evaluators concluded that more studies were needed focusing on "consistent administration and reproducible dosing of marijuana, potentially through the use of administration methods other than smoking" [28]. Additionally, although dronabinol and nabilone had been approved for 30 years by 2015, there were no FDA-approved cannabis-derived products or any cannabis products under a new drug application (NDA) or biologics license application for any indication, a key component in proving a drug is accepted by qualified experts (according to the FDA) [27]. Here's what's happened in the intervening years to refute these concerns:

6.3.1   Continued Research in the Field of Cannabis Medicine

In the most recent HHS assessment, evaluators concluded that the five-part CAMU test was insufficient because it did not provide flexibility to account for the widespread medical use of cannabis outside the realm of FDA-approved substances. In 2017, the NASEM systematic review concluded that there was substantial evidence supporting the use of cannabinoids to treat chronic pain and muscle spasms associated with MS and moderate evidence supporting the use of cannabinoids in the treatment of insomnia [29]. NASEM advises the US government on matters of science and technology; its founding organization, the National Academy of Sciences, was established by Congress in 1863 [30]. Clinical investigations into the therapeutic uses of cannabis continue despite the challenges in conducting such research in the United States. In 2023, the NIH supported 222 investigations into cannabinoid therapeutics with over $127 million in funding [31]. In its 2023 report, HHS concluded that, on balance, medical research shows that cannabis has value as a treatment for chronic pain, anorexia associated with a medical condition, and nausea and vomiting.

6.3.2   Approval of a Botanical Cannabis Extract

One of the most momentous recent developments in cannabis medicine was the approval of plant-derived CBD in 2018. Although synthetic cannabinoids had previously been approved, they were not considered sufficient evidence by the FDA to support the claim that the cannabis plant had an accepted medical use. Purified CBD, extracted from greenhouse-grown cannabis plants, is approved for the treatment of three severe seizure disorders that primarily affect children [32]. The USP is drafting an official monograph for CBD [33] and has also proposed a monograph for the cannabis plant [34]. Once approved, cannabis will be back in the USP after almost 90 years.

6.3.3   The Modern Cannabis Market Is So Much More than Joints and Bongs

Although smoking dried cannabis flower has historically been the preferred method of administration, the cannabis industry has introduced new formulations, many of which do not need to be inhaled via smoking or vaporization. These include food products ("edibles"), tinctures, oromucosal sprays, topical or transdermal preparations, and suppositories [35]. An Israeli company has developed a metered-dose inhaler for cannabis products that allows for uniform dosing; this option may be helpful in patients for whom the rapid onset of action associated with inhalation is important (e.g., cancer pain), without the pulmonary adverse effects associated with smoking [36].

6.3.4   Big Pharma's Growing (Pun Intended) Interest in Cannabinoid Products

Ease of research may encourage greater participation by the global pharmaceutical industry, which has by and large been a spectator thus far in the bourgeoning cannabis industry. There's no doubt that the cannabis industry is lucrative; in 2022, the US cannabis market was valued at \$13.2 billion and is expected to grow at a rate of about 14% per year [37]. For years, the pharmaceutical industry has devoted "substantial lobbying efforts and resources" to oppose cannabis legalization in the United States, probably due to concerns that patients might opt to manage medical conditions with legal cannabis rather than using traditional pharmaceutical treatments [38]. A 2022 study indicated that legalizing cannabis entirely (i.e., removing it from the CSA) could result in the loss of billions of dollars in stock market returns for pharmaceutical companies [39]. Rescheduling cannabis might not have the same effect but, instead, make it easier for pharmaceutical companies (who have more resources for navigating the drug development process with the FDA than smaller cannabis companies) to develop and profit from new medical cannabis products.

6.4   What Does a Federal Cannabis Program Look like?

Even with rescheduling in the works (at the time of this writing), there will still be many questions about federal medical cannabis policy moving forward. Unlike other Schedule I substances, many states have a thriving cannabis industry, each with its own policies and regulations. The cannabis products currently consumed by patients are (as previously mentioned) not approved by the FDA. It's unlikely, though not impossible, that most cannabis companies will engage in a lengthy and costly drug approval process for products that can already be sold on the state market. Will there be an alternative process for providing FDA oversight of these products? If not, we should expect that states will continue to regulate their own medical cannabis markets rather than attempt to conform to federal law. Non-medical state cannabis markets will, of course, be unaffected by rescheduling. Other questions include whether the FDA will be able to cope with the influx of applications if rescheduling does lead to a flood of research, development, investigational new drug applications, and NDAs related to medical cannabis products and whether the FDA will develop additional guidance and standards for cultivation, processing, and analytical testing of cannabis plants and products.

6.5   That's Rescheduling—What About Descheduling?

Many advocates for cannabis reform oppose rescheduling in favor of removing cannabis from regulation under the CSA altogether and regulating it like alcohol or tobacco. This would have many implications for the cannabis industry and social reform. However, "descheduling" would not reflect an acknowledgment of cannabis as medicine, and likely, medical cannabis would be relegated to the fringe of Western medicine along with other complementary and alternative treatments. Although fully legalizing cannabis could improve access for some patients, cannabis companies would largely focus on developing products likely to be popular with non-medical users, the larger consumer population.

References

1. Griffin R, Swetlitz I, Kary T. US health officials urge moving pot to lower-risk tier. Bloomberg. 2023. https://www.bloomberg.com/news/articles/2023-08-30/hhs-calls-for-moving-marijuana-to-lower-risk-us-drug-category. Accessed 28 Aug 2024.
2. U.S. Drug Enforcement Administration. Drug scheduling. 2018. https://www.dea.gov/drug-information/drug-scheduling. Accessed 28 Aug 2024
3. Bonini SA, Premoli M, Tambaro S, et al. Cannabis sativa: a comprehensive ethnopharmacological review of a medicinal plant with a long history. J Ethnopharmacol. 2018;227:300–15. https://doi.org/10.1016/j.jep.2018.09.004.
4. Atkins P. Everything old is new again: cannabis returns to USP. Cannab Sci Technol. 2020;3(5):17–22. https://www.cannabissciencetech.com/view/everything-old-new-again-cannabis-returns-usp. Accessed 28 Aug 2024.
5. Pisanti S, Bifulco M. Modern history of medical cannabis: from widespread use to prohibitionism and back. Trends Pharmacol Sci. 2017;38(3):195–8. https://doi.org/10.1016/j.tips.2016.12.002.
6. Hudak J. Marijuana: a short history. 2nd ed. Brookings Institution Press; 2020.
7. LaGuardia F. The LaGuardia committee report: the marihuana problem in the City of New York (NY). Mayor's committee on marihuana (US); 1941. https://rodneybarnett.net/PDF/Laguardia%20Report%201944.pdf.
8. United Nations. United Nations conference for the adoption of a single convention on narcotic drugs 24 January–25 March 1961, N Y; 1961. https://www.un.org/en/conferences/drug/newyork1961. Accessed Aug 30 2024.
9. Gabay M. The Federal Controlled Substances act: schedules and pharmacy registration. Hosp Pharm. 2013;48(6):473. https://doi.org/10.1310/HPJ4806-473.
10. NORML. A brief history of cannabis rescheduling petitions in the United States. Fact Sheets. https://norml.org/marijuana/fact-sheets/a-brief-history-of-cannabis-rescheduling-petitions-in-the-united-states/. Accessed Aug 30 2024.
11. Zeese KB. History of medical marijuana policy in US. Int J Drug Policy. 1999;10:319–28. www.csdp.org. Accessed 2024 Aug 30.

12. National Conference of state legislatures. State medical cannabis Laws. 2023. https://www.ncsl.org/health/state-medical-cannabis-laws. Accessed Aug 30 2024.
13. Felson J, Adamczyk A, Thomas C. How and why have attitudes about cannabis legalization changed so much? Soc Sci Res. 2019;78:12–27. https://doi.org/10.1016/J.SSRESEARCH.2018.12.011.
14. Ogden DW. Memorandum for selected united state attorneys on investigations and prosecutions in states authorizing the medical use of marijuana. United States Department of Justice Archives. 2009. https://www.justice.gov/archives/opa/blog/memorandum-selected-united-state-attorneys-investigations-and-prosecutions-states. Accessed 2024 Aug 30.
15. Roman ZS. Tenth Circuit decision clears the way for further judicial consideration of application of recently re-enacted Rohrabacher-Farr Amendment. Reed Smith Client Alerts. 2019. https://www.reedsmith.com/en/perspectives/2019/12/tenth-circuit-decision-clears-the-way-for-further-judicial-consideration. Accessed 30 Aug 2024.
16. Volkow ND. The overdose crisis: interagency proposal to combat illicit fentanyl-related substances. Presented at: 2021 Dec 2. https://nida.nih.gov/about-nida/legislative-activities/testimony-to-congress/2021/the-overdose-crisis-proposal-to-combat-illicit-fentanyl. Accessed Aug 30 2024.
17. Milgram A. O'Malley KN. Prevoznik TW. Valentine NS. Drug Enforcement Administration Researcher's Manual. DEA Diversion Control Division. Revised 2022. https://www.deadiversion.usdoj.gov/GDP/(DEA-DC-057)(EO-DEA217)_Researchers_Manual_Final_signed.pdf. Accessed 30 Aug 2024.
18. Kaylor A. How regulation stymies medical research of controlled substances. PharmaNews Intelligence 2022. https://pharmanewsintel.com/features/barriers-to-medical-research-constructed-by-federally-controlled-substance-scheduling-and-classification. Accessed Aug 30 2024.
19. Rønne ST, Rosenbæk F, Pedersen LB, et al. Physicians' experiences, attitudes, and beliefs towards medical cannabis: a systematic literature review. BMC Fam Pract. 2021;22(1):212. https://doi.org/10.1186/s12875-021-01559-w.
20. Americans for Safe Access. 2022 State of the states report: an analysis of medical cannabis access in the United States. 2022. https://www.safeaccessnow.org/sos22. Accessed Aug 30 2024.
21. Drug Enforcement Administration. FDA-approved drug Epidiolex placed in schedule V of Controlled Substance Act. 2018. https://www.dea.gov/press-releases/2018/09/27/fda-approved-drug-epidiolex-placed-schedule-v-controlled-substance-act. Accessed Aug 30.
22. DEA Deschedules antiepileptic CBD Oral solution Epidiolex. Drug Topics 2020. https://www.drugtopics.com/view/dea-deschedules-antiepileptic-cbd-oral-solution-epidiolex. Accessed Aug 30 2024.

23. Hudak J. The farm bill, hemp legalization and the status of CBD: an explainer. Brookings institution Commentary. 2018. https://www.brookings.edu/articles/the-farm-bill-hemp-and-cbd-explainer/. Accessed Aug 30 2024.

24. Internal revenue code 280E: creating an impossible situation for legitimate businesses. National Cannabis Industry Association. 2015. https://thecannabisindustry.org/reports/internal-revenue-code-280e-creating-an-impossible-situation-for-legitimate-businesses/. Accessed Aug 30 2024.

25. What is 280E? [Internet] Marijuana Policy Project. Available from: https://www.mpp.org/policy/federal/what-is-280e/. Accessed Aug 30 2024.

26. Biden J. Statement from president Biden on marijuana reform. White House Briefing Room Statement and Releases. 2022. https://www.whitehouse.gov/briefing-room/statements-releases/2022/10/06/statement-from-president-biden-on-marijuana-reform/. Accessed 2024 Aug 30.

27. Drug Enforcement Administration. Denial of petition to initiate proceedings to reschedule marijuana. Fed Regist. 2016;1:53688–766.

28. Bonner RC. Marijuana scheduling petition; denial of petition. Remand Fed Regist. 1992;57(59):10499–508.

29. National Academies of Sciences, Engineering, and Medicine. The health effects of cannabis and cannabinoids: the current state of evidence and recommendations for research. The National Academies Press; 2017. https://doi.org/10.17226/24625.

30. National Academy of Sciences. About NAS: Founding and Early Work [Internet]. https://www.nasonline.org/about-nas/history/archives/founding-and-early-work.html. Accessed Aug 30 2024.

31. National Center for Complementary and Integrative Health. NIH-supported research on cannabis, cannabinoids, and related compounds. 2023. https://www.nccih.nih.gov/grants/nih-supported-research-on-cannabis-cannabinoids-and-related-compounds. Accessed Aug 30 2024.

32. Abu-Sawwa R, Scutt B, Park Y. Emerging use of Epidiolex (cannabidiol) in epilepsy. J Pediatr Pharmacol Ther. 2020;25(6):485–99. https://doi.org/10.5863/1551-6776-25.6.485.

33. USP draft monograph for CBD. ECA Academy. 2022. https://www.gmp-compliance.org/gmp-news/usp-draft-monograph-for-cbd. Accessed Aug 30 2024.

34. Roussel C, Schwartz M. USP, FDA propose quality standards for cannabis, highlighting its role as medicine. Pharm Times. 2023. https://www.pharmacytimes.com/view/usp-fda-propose-quality-standards-for-cannabis-highlighting-its-role-as-medicine. Accessed Aug 30 2024.

35. Spindle TR, Bonn-Miller MO, Vandrey R. Changing landscape of cannabis: novel products, formulations, and methods of administration. Curr Opin Psychol. 2019;30:98–102. https://doi.org/10.1016/j.copsyc.2019.04.002.

36. SyqueAir. SyqeAir Cannabis Inhaler [Internet]. https://syqe.com/air-by-syqe-inhaler/. Accessed Aug 30 2024.

37. U.S. Cannabis Market Size, Share & Trends Report U.S. Cannabis Market Size, Share & Trends Analysis Report By End-use (Medical, Recreational, Industrial), By Source (Marijuana, Hemp), By Derivative (CBD, THC), And Segment Forecasts, 2023–2030. Grand View Research. 2023. https://www.grandviewresearch.com/industry-analysis/us-cannabis-market. Accessed 2024 Aug 30.
38. Jaeger K. Pharmaceutical industry suffers billions in losses after states legalize marijuana, new study finds. Marijuana Moment. 2022. https://www.marijuanamoment.net/pharmaceutical-industry-suffers-billions-in-losses-after-states-legalize-marijuana-new-study-finds/. Accessed Aug 30 2024.
39. Bednarek Z, Doremus JM, Stith SS. U.S. cannabis laws projected to cost generic and brand pharmaceutical firms billions. PLoS One. 2022;17(8 August):e0272492. https://doi.org/10.1371/journal.pone.0272492.

A Modern Clinician's Approach to the Medical Cannabis Era

7

7.1 The Clinician's Role in Medical Cannabis Care

This chapter is the "meat and potatoes" of medical cannabis care for the modern clinician. It will provide insight and discussion of common concerns and potential myths about providing medical cannabis education or care to patients. It will explore the common concerns about risks, including the risk of addiction, psychosis, cannabis use during pregnancy, and other vulnerable patient groups. A proposed approach to a medical visit with a patient interested in using medical cannabis is included, along with language for safe counseling and education.

The modern clinician faces many new challenges as patient access to cannabis products expands across the country. Patients of all ages have increasing awareness of the availability of cannabis and the growing body of anecdotal and clinical evidence. The legal landscape at the state level diverges from current federal laws regulating cannabis, resulting in confusion, stigma, and a persistent disconnect between clinicians and patients. One of the biggest challenges that modern clinicians must overcome is a worldview in which patients using cannabis for symptom relief have substance use disorder. Instead, the modern clinician should adopt an approach that recognizes the potential for cannabis as a

L. Sera, C. Hempel-Sanderoff, *Cannabis Science and Therapeutics*, https://doi.org/10.1007/978-3-031-80352-9_7

legitimate medical therapy and acknowledges many patients' desire for a more patient-driven or shared decision-making approach to health and wellness.

Knowledge and practice gaps are significant among many clinicians in primary care. In surveys, clinicians often state that they believe that medical cannabis has potential medical benefits and believe it is helpful for conditions such as cancer and chronic pain, with up to 60% supporting its legalization [1]. And yet, only 20–30% of clinicians believed that family physicians and primary care providers should recommend the use of cannabis [2]. These conflicting viewpoints and practice patterns present ongoing challenges as the cannabis landscape shifts from "illicit drug use" to "accepted medical use." At the time of this writing, an estimated 35 million people in the United States report using cannabis, with more than 78 million reporting lifetime cannabis use [3]. An estimated three million people report using cannabis for symptom relief and chronic illness [4]. It is time for clinicians to adapt their clinical approach to the patient interested in or using medical cannabis.

This chapter will explore some of the main concerns of clinicians regarding medical cannabis and will hopefully help provide a more secure and comfortable approach to the growing prevalence of patient cannabis access. The concerns below will be addressed:

1. Will I lose my license for discussing cannabis with my patients?
2. What is the difference between "prescribing" and "recommending" cannabis?
3. What risks are associated with medical cannabis use, and how can I reduce potential harm for my patients who use medical cannabis?

7.2   Will I Lose My License for Discussing Cannabis with my Patients?

The short answer is no. This may be one of the biggest cannabis-related misconceptions made by clinicians today, and dispelling this myth is essential to the forward progress of the field of cannabis medicine. The clinician-patient relationship is protected under the First Amendment, which supports unrestricted communication necessary to ensure appropriate patient care, with legal precedent from the US Court of Appeals [5]. The practical application of this ruling protects the role of the clinician as teacher and counselor regarding medical cannabis. It is perfectly legal for clinicians to discuss cannabis science and evidence, common cannabis formulations, and potential risks and monitor privately with their patients. Having said that, there are many institutions that prohibit employed clinicians from engaging financially with the cannabis industry or conducting cannabis research. Institutions and health systems that rely on federal funding may adopt a conservative approach to medical cannabis, given the current Schedule I status of cannabis, regardless of state laws.

In states where cannabis is legal and if their employer allows it, physicians may recommend medical cannabis for specific patients if they believe it may be helpful for a certain condition [6]. A simpler way to look at it is this: it is perfectly legal to talk about or teach about medical cannabis and associated topics (like the ECS). Clinicians who facilitate the sale of cannabis, for instance, by owning a dispensary or who conduct cannabis research without proper licensing and regulatory approval could be considered "aiding and abetting" the distribution of a controlled substance [5].

7.3 What Is the Difference Between "Prescribing" and "Recommending" Medical Cannabis?

This common misuse of terminology is widespread among clinicians and patients alike. In the United States, it is illegal to *prescribe* any drug designated as a Schedule I substance, including cannabis products. Therefore, except for the few FDA-approved cannabinoid products on the market (dronabinol, nabilone, and CBD oil), it is incorrect to state that clinicians *prescribe* medical cannabis for patients. The accurate terminology, which highlights the correct legal practice, is that clinicians *recommend* medical cannabis for patients. A licensed physician in any US state (whether cannabis is legal or not) may decide to suggest or recommend medical cannabis based on their clinical judgment and expertise. In states that have an established medical cannabis program, it is also legal for physicians to facilitate patient access to medical cannabis in accordance with state regulations by *certifying* that they have a medical condition that may benefit from medical cannabis use [6].

7.4   What Risks Are Associated with Medical Cannabis Use, and How Can I Reduce Potential Harm for my Patients Who Use Medical Cannabis?

While there are few absolute contraindications (such as an allergy to cannabis or components of a cannabis product) to the use of medical cannabis, increased risk does exist for some vulnerable populations. The modern clinician should be able to identify areas of vulnerability and patients for whom cannabis use may be harmful, as well as monitor for adverse effects in patients for whom medical cannabis is an appropriate therapeutic option. This section describes precautions to consider when recommending medical cannabis and the possible adverse effects of THC and CBD.

7.4.1   Risk of Cannabis Use Disorder

A major concern regarding medical cannabis use is the risk of aberrant use or addiction. Since cannabis is currently designated as a Schedule I substance, many clinicians perceive that cannabis is highly addictive with little medical utility. The definition of a Schedule I drug is a drug that is considered to have the highest likelihood of abuse and no currently accepted medical use, so this perception is unsurprising. In recent years, large population studies and data from the National Institute on Drug Abuse have more clearly delineated the prevalence of CUD. CUD develops in an estimated 5–10% of all cannabis users and manifests similarly to other substance use disorders [7]. Daily cannabis users can experience withdrawal symptoms, including irritability, insomnia, and mood fluctuations, when they discontinue use [8]. CUD is more likely when a person continues to use cannabis despite negative physical, emotional, or social consequences. Daily use of high-potency cannabis appears to increase the risk of dependence and CUD significantly [9, 10]. CUD is also discussed in Sect. 5.2.

Harm Reduction Tip
- Recommend CBD-only products preferentially for patients with a history of SUD/CUD or who are at high risk of developing CUD.
- At each visit, discuss cannabinoid dosage and use patterns and ask about negative social or psychological effects.
- If concerns for CUD arise, discuss them directly with the patient, offer support, and address any referrals needed.

7.4.2   Risk of Psychosis

The psychoactive effects of THC produce progressive impairment that is dose-dependent and produces temporary intoxication in most users. In a subset of vulnerable people, this intoxication can result in temporary or permanent psychosis. While the overall reported prevalence is low (0.47% of cannabis users who sought medical attention in one large study presented with psychotic symptoms), the lifelong consequences and functional impairment resulting from cannabis-induced psychosis can be devastating [11]. Recent studies have helped to identify those at increased risk for first-episode psychosis, which includes those with prior diagnoses of psychosis, schizophrenia, and bipolar disorder or family histories of these diagnoses, suggesting a genetic predisposition that warrants further research [12]. Males who use cannabis at a young age with frequent (i.e., daily) use and/or who use high-potency cannabis products appear to be at greater risk for developing psychosis [13].

Harm Reduction Tip
- Counsel all medical cannabis patients about the increased risk of psychosis with daily use of high-potency THC products. Advise patients to avoid cannabis vape oil and cannabis concentrates, especially adolescent males.

- Screen for patient and family history of schizophrenia, bipolar disorder, or psychosis. If present, advise against THC use and recommend CBD-only products.

7.4.3 Cannabis Use During Pregnancy

Many women believe cannabis use is safe during pregnancy, and recent studies indicate that about 30–60% of cannabis users plan to continue use during pregnancy, with an estimated prevalence of cannabis use in 2–5% of pregnancies [14]. Cannabis use appears to have a negative effect on pregnancy outcomes, including greater odds of pre-term birth, small-for-gestational-age size, and perinatal mortality [15]. THC crosses the placental barrier and can impact fetal ECS signaling that regulates neuron development in key brain structures, including the hippocampus and forebrain [16]. Notably, infants born in the setting of cannabis use appear to have stronger startle reflexes, more fragmented sleep cycles, and increased body movements [17, 18]. The long-term effects of these findings continue to be the subject of intense research, with questions about the impact on cognition and psychological health later in life. Cannabis use during pregnancy is also discussed in Sect. 6.4. For now, the harm-reductive approach for clinicians is to counsel any pregnant patient about the risks of cannabis use and to recommend abstaining from cannabis use during pregnancy.

7.4.4 Cannabis Use in Patients of Advanced Age

One of the fastest-growing groups of patients exploring medical cannabis is the senior population (age 65+). Common conditions for which these patients seek medical cannabis are similar to other age groups—chronic non-cancer pain, cancer pain, anxiety, insomnia, and diminished appetite [19]. This group requires more attention as they are more likely to have multiple comorbid conditions, degenerative diseases, cognitive impairment, medical frailty, and polypharmacy. Alterations in metabolism can produce unpredictable or paradoxical effects in this age group, requiring closer monitoring. Potential risks of cannabis use in the elderly are similar to other psychoactive medications and include dizziness, hypotension, impaired balance and falls, cognitive and memory impairment, sedation, or paradoxical agitation [20].

Harm Reduction Tip
- Recommend no THC or very low THC products, with a focus on CBD preferentially.
- Start with the lowest doses and titrate slowly.
- Counsel family and caregivers about safety, storage, and signs of intoxication.
- Need for increased frequency of monitoring in patients at risk of drug interactions (see Chap. 8, Table 8.8).

7.4.5   Cannabis Use in Pediatric Patients

The pediatric population represents a uniquely vulnerable group. Age, cognitive development, and the severity of childhood illness all limit the ability of patients to make informed decisions for themselves. Hence, pediatric patients rely on parents or caregivers to protect their well-being and best interests. Few RCTs have evaluated cannabinoids in pediatric patients; nabilone and dronabinol have demonstrated effectiveness in improving chemotherapy-induced nausea and vomiting compared to placebo in children, and CBD oil has demonstrated effectiveness in treating drug-resistant epilepsy [21]. For other conditions, evidence is scant, low-quality, or based entirely on preclinical data, creating an ethical and morally challenging space for patients, caregivers, providers, and researchers. Additionally, there are legal implications, as state laws vary regarding certifying and administering cannabinoids for minors. For example, some states require a two-physician certification, and several require specific certification from a pediatrician and a psychiatrist for registering pediatric patients in medical cannabis programs.

Most studies of cannabis risk in pediatric populations evaluated non-medical cannabis use, and very few included children under 10 years old. Risks are directly related to THC concentration and include decreased motivation, addiction, schizophrenia, and mild cognitive decline [22]. Until more is known about the short- and long-term risks of altering the developing ECS, consideration of medical cannabis in children should be limited to severe, refractory, or life-limiting conditions as part of a shared decision-making process with parents, pediatricians, and specialists.

7.5   Essential Components of a Medical Cannabis Visit

Optimal care for patients using medical cannabis requires an individualized approach, addressing each patient's unique conditions, symptoms, risks, cannabis use history, and preferences. In states with established medical cannabis programs, after obtaining a history and examining the patient, clinicians can certify that a patient has a medical condition that may be improved by using medical cannabis (called a *qualifying condition*). This certification is submitted to the state cannabis program, and a medical cannabis registration identification card is usually issued to the patient, which allows them to enter a dispensary and purchase cannabis products. The *certification* serves as an attestation that the patient has the qualifying conditions listed in that state's medical cannabis program regulations. Since the details and requirements of state programs are highly variable with ongoing changes, clinicians should check with their state cannabis regulatory agency for guidance on participating as a certifying provider.

Outside of this setting, an increasing number of primary care providers, specialists, and pharmacists are encountering patients with questions about cannabis or with an interest in using medical cannabis for symptoms or chronic health conditions. In the past, cannabis users were assumed to have a substance use disorder, and the approach of many clinicians has been either to discourage use universally or to avoid the subject. Since public perception regarding use is evolving, with use becoming more widely accepted and cannabis becoming increasingly accessible to the general public, supporting patients as they explore and integrate cannabis with their other treatments and medications is an important role of the modern clinician. Below, we provide an outline that includes essential elements of a visit with a patient regarding medical cannabis use (Table 7.1).

Table 7.1 Components of a medical cannabis clinical encounter [23]

Component	Comment
Chief complaint	The primary reason for the clinical encounter
Complete medical and surgical history	This is standard practice for any history and physical or consultation
Mental health history (personal and family)	An essential component of medical cannabis care is to identify risks or potential contraindications. Personal histories or family histories of psychosis, bipolar disorder, or CUD may be poor candidates for medical cannabis or require close monitoring
History of present illness and symptom analysis	Identify and describe the specific symptoms for which the patient is seeking relief using medical cannabis. This will inform a review of medical literature in preparation for informed discussion and counseling
Medications (prescription, nonprescription, vitamins/supplements)	A complete review of current medications and supplements is necessary to assess the potential for drug-drug interactions and determine if specialized monitoring is needed
Prior cannabis use	This is very helpful for identifying the patient's prior response to cannabis (THC in particular). This can guide recommendations for selecting the ideal cannabinoid ratio to optimize therapeutic benefits and minimize adverse effects. It can also help with identifying the patient's preferred formulation
Patient treatment goals and indices of efficacy	Patient goals for therapy should be individualized based on the presenting symptoms. Complete relief may not be possible, so establishing goals is helpful to measure improvement over time. Examples of specific goals could be: • Pain scale reduction from 8 to 4 on a scale of 0 to 10 • Enough improvement in nausea to be able to eat a meal • Enough improvement in anxiety to be able to sleep through the night or attend a social event

(continued)

Table 7.1 (continued)

Component	Comment
Identify the ideal cannabinoid ratio	In general, type II (balanced THC/CBD) or type III cannabinoids (CBD-dominant) are recommended for medical use in most patients
Identify preferred formulation	Once the ideal cannabinoid ratio is selected, the preferred formulation is then identified by the patient due to their individual situation and goals Lung health, cannabis palatability, dexterity, visual limitations, potential impairment, and prior effects all influence the selection of the ideal cannabis formulation for individual patients
Monitoring and follow-up	Follow up every 1–2 weeks for new medical cannabis patients. The follow-up period can be extended to monthly or bi-monthly once the dose and symptoms stabilize. After 6 months, the follow-up interval can be determined by the patient and clinician, with a minimum of one follow-up visit every 6 months Monitoring should include screening for: • Symptom relief or worsening • Current dosing and formulation (red flag if daily THC dose >40 mg) • Adverse effects • New problems or symptoms • New medications • Indications of CUD or substance abuse • Patient global perception of effectiveness and progress toward treatment goals
Communication with other providers	Collaborating with the patient's care team about medical cannabis treatment helps ensure high-quality overall care With the patient's permission, sending a brief letter or consultation note to other involved providers can help unify the care team and reduce fragmentation of care This practice can help overcome stigma and educate other clinicians about medical cannabis and clinical evidence

7.6   Language for Safe Counseling

Many clinicians express concern about the purported legal risk of discussing or recommending medical cannabis to patients. It is a common misconception that clinicians are forbidden to consider the potential therapeutic properties of cannabis due to its current Schedule I status. However, with the intentional use of appropriate terminology and language, clinicians can safely discuss cannabis science, therapeutic properties, common cannabis formulations, risks, and evidence with patients. Given the dearth of clinical evidence for cannabis therapy in many disease states and the lack of disease-specific guidelines, clinicians cannot reasonably state that "cannabis is safe and effective for condition X." How, then, do we support and counsel patients appropriately? Below, we propose some specific language that may help guide clinicians and increase comfort around discussing medical cannabis. Adapt these statements to the relevant conditions, patient scenarios, and available medical evidence.

Recommended Language for Patient Counseling
- "Patients tend to report relief or improvement from this symptom with the use of medical cannabis."
- "It is still too early to say definitively whether medical cannabis is helpful for this symptom, but preclinical research and patient reports seem to suggest a benefit."
- "Our understanding of the role of medical cannabis is limited in this condition, but your persistent symptoms, despite trying other traditional treatments, make a trial of medical cannabis reasonable in this situation."
- "I can't say definitively whether cannabis is effective or whether the products at the dispensary are the same as the studies. The low-risk approach appears to be a trial of low-dose THC with higher amounts of CBD for most conditions."
- "Medical cannabis still has risks despite being legal in this state, and the products are not approved or regulated

by the FDA. I encourage you to look for formulations that have very little THC with higher proportions of CBD."

- "There are no specific recommendations or guidelines for using medical cannabis in the treatment of this condition, but small clinical trials suggest that THC doses of 2–5 mg daily, and CBD doses of 20–40 mg daily have shown some benefit."

Language to Avoid
- "Medical cannabis is great for this condition."
- "I will prescribe medical cannabis for your chronic pain."
- "Cannabis is illegal, and I am not allowed to discuss it."
- "Studies prove that medical cannabis treats this condition."
- "There is no evidence for medical cannabis use, so I won't discuss it."

After digesting all the science, evidence, and clinical information in the first eight chapters, the next question on your mind is likely "What does this look like in real life?" In Chap. 9, we will explore some case studies to illustrate how the modern clinician might approach a typical medical cannabis patient visit. We hope you will feel more comfortable and confident in your ability to offer high-quality and compassionate medical cannabis care!

References

1. Philpot LM, Ebbert JO, Hurt RT. A survey of the attitudes, beliefs and knowledge about medical cannabis among primary care providers. BMC Fam Pract. 2019;20(1):17. https://doi.org/10.1186/s12875-019-0906-y. PMID: 30669979; PMCID: PMC6341534.
2. Abo Ziad R, Grynbaum MB, Peleg R, Treister-Goltzman Y. The attitudes and beliefs of family physicians regarding the use of medical cannabis, knowledge of side effects, and barriers to use: a comparison between residents and specialists. Am J Ther. 2022;29(4):e400–9. https://doi.org/10.1097/MJT.0000000000001236.
3. National Center for Drug Abuse Statistics. Marijuana addiction: rates and usage statistics [Internet]. 2024. https://drugabusestatistics.org/marijuana-addiction/#. Accessed 4 Sep 2024
4. Ryan JE, McCabe SE, Boyd CJ. Medicinal cannabis: policy, patients, and providers. Policy Polit Nurs Pract. 2021;22(2):126–33. https://doi.org/10.1177/1527154421989609. Epub 2021 Feb 10. PMID: 33567970; PMCID: PMC8098049.
5. Gregorio J. Physicians, medical marijuana, and the law. Virtual Mentor. 2014;16(9):732–8. https://doi.org/10.1001/virtualmentor.2014.16.09.hlaw1-1409.
6. National Conference of State Legislatures. Medical uses of cannabis [Internet]. Updated 2024 Jul 12. https://www.ncsl.org/health/state-medical-cannabis-laws. Accessed Sep 4 2024.
7. Connor JP, Stjepanović D, Le Foll B, Hoch E, Budney AJ, Hall WD. Cannabis use and cannabis use disorder. Nat Rev Dis Primers. 2021;7(1):16. https://doi.org/10.1038/s41572-021-00247-4. PMID: 33627670; PMCID: PMC8655458.
8. Connor JP, Stjepanović D, Budney AJ, Le Foll B, Hall WD. Clinical management of cannabis withdrawal. Addiction. 2022;117(7):2075–95. https://doi.org/10.1111/add.15743. Epub 2022 Jan 10. PMID: 34791767; PMCID: PMC9110555.
9. Petrilli K, Ofori S, Hines L, Taylor G, Adams S, Freeman TP. Association of cannabis potency with mental ill health and addiction: a systematic review. Lancet Psychiatry. 2022;9(9):736–50. https://doi.org/10.1016/S2215-0366(22)00161-4. Epub 2022 Jul 25.
10. Robinson T, Ali MU, Easterbrook B, Coronado-Montoya S, Daldegan-Bueno D, Hall W, Jutras-Aswad D, Fischer B. Identifying risk-thresholds for the association between frequency of cannabis use and development of cannabis use disorder: a systematic review and meta-analysis. Drug Alcohol Depend. 2022;238:109582. https://doi.org/10.1016/j.drugalcdep.2022.109582. Epub 2022 Jul 21.
11. Schoeler T, Ferris J, Winstock AR. Rates and correlates of cannabis-associated psychotic symptoms in over 230,000 people who use cannabis.

Transl Psychiatry. 2022;12(1):369. https://doi.org/10.1038/s41398-022-02112-8. PMID: 36068202; PMCID: PMC9448725.

12. Carvalho C, Vieira-Coelho MA. Cannabis induced psychosis: a systematic review on the role of genetic polymorphisms. Pharmacol Res. 2022;181:106258. https://doi.org/10.1016/j.phrs.2022.106258. Epub 2022 May 16.

13. Di Forti M, Marconi A, Carra E, Fraietta S, Trotta A, Bonomo M, Bianconi F, Gardner-Sood P, O'Connor J, Russo M, Stilo SA, Marques TR, Mondelli V, Dazzan P, Pariante C, David AS, Gaughran F, Atakan Z, Iyegbe C, Powell J, Morgan C, Lynskey M, Murray RM. Proportion of patients in South London with first-episode psychosis attributable to use of high potency cannabis: a case-control study. Lancet Psychiatry. 2015;2(3):233–8. https://doi.org/10.1016/S2215-0366(14)00117-5. Epub 2015 Feb 25.

14. Lo JO, Shaw B, Robalino S, Ayers CK, Durbin S, Rushkin MC, Olyaei A, Kansagara D, Harrod CS. Cannabis use in pregnancy and neonatal outcomes: a systematic review and meta-analysis. Cannabis Cannabinoid Res. 2024;9(2):470–85. https://doi.org/10.1089/can.2022.0262. Epub 2023 Feb 1. PMID: 36730710; PMCID: PMC11262585.

15. Baía I, Domingues RMSM. The effects of cannabis use during pregnancy on low birth weight and preterm birth: a systematic review and meta-analysis. Am J Perinatol. 2024;41(1):17–30. https://doi.org/10.1055/a-1911-3326. Epub 2022 Jul 28.

16. Abrams RM, Cook CE, Davis KH, Niederreither K, Jaeger MJ, Szeto HH. Plasma delta-9-tetrahydrocannabinol in pregnant sheep and fetus after inhalation of smoke from a marijuana cigarette. Alcohol. Drug Res. 1985–1986;6(5):361–9.

17. Berghuis P, Rajnicek AM, Morozov YM, Ross RA, Mulder J, Urbán GM, Monory K, Marsicano G, Matteoli M, Canty A, Irving AJ, Katona I, Yanagawa Y, Rakic P, Lutz B, Mackie K, Harkany T. Hardwiring the brain: endocannabinoids shape neuronal connectivity. Science. 2007;316(5828):1212–6. https://doi.org/10.1126/science.1137406.

18. Cristino L, Di Marzo V. Fetal cannabinoid receptors and the "dis-jointed" brain. EMBO J. 2014;33(7):665–7. https://doi.org/10.1002/embj.201488086. Epub 2014 Mar 14. PMID: 24631837; PMCID: PMC4000085.

19. Abuhasira R, Schleider LB, Mechoulam R, Novack V. Epidemiological characteristics, safety and efficacy of medical cannabis in the elderly. Eur J Intern Med. 2018;49:44–50. https://doi.org/10.1016/j.ejim.2018.01.019.

20. Nathan R, Mupamombe CT, Elibol J, Case AA, Smith D, Hyland A, Attwood K, Hansen ED. Assessing efficacy and use patterns of medical cannabis for symptom management in elderly cancer patients. Am J Hosp Palliat Care. 2023;40(4):368–73. https://doi.org/10.1177/10499091221110217. Epub 2022 Jun 24.

21. Treves N, Mor N, Allegaert K, Bassalov H, Berkovitch M, Stolar OE, et al. Efficacy and safety of medical cannabinoids in children: a systematic review and meta-analysis. Sci Rep. 2021;11(1):23462–11.
22. Aran A, Cayam-Rand D. Medical cannabis in children. Rambam Maimonides Med J. 2020;11(1):e0003.
23. Khazen M, Sullivan EE, Ramos J, Mirica M, Linzer M, Schiff GD, Olson APJ. Anatomy of diagnosis in a clinical encounter: how clinicians discuss uncertainty with patients. BMC Prim Care. 2022;23(1):153. https://doi.org/10.1186/s12875-022-01767-y. PMID: 35715733; PMCID: PMC9205543.

Practical Matters: Cannabis Formulations and Dosing

8

In this chapter, we outline an approach to the initial dosing and selection of medical cannabis formulations for different groups of patients. There are currently no disease-specific dosing recommendations, so a patient-specific approach to dosing is the current practice. The overwhelming variety of medical cannabis formulations and their effects are defined for quick reference. An outline for dosing, titration, monitoring, and discontinuation is provided for cannabis-naive patients, experienced patients, and patients with severe symptoms. Considerations about drug interactions, monitoring, and adverse effects are also provided.

8.1 A Word About Modern Cannabis Potency

In this chapter, we will explore the numerous cannabis formulations that are currently available to medical cannabis patients. Before proceeding, we need to provide some context regarding an important factor in the evolution of cannabis cultivation over the past several decades. In the 1960s, the average THC potency in botanical cannabis plants was less than 10%. Modern cannabis plants are significantly more potent, with THC concentrations averaging closer to 12–15% [1]. It is not uncommon to find cannabis flower containing 30% THC or higher in state dispensaries. In addition, high-potency cannabis extracts and concentrates can

© The Author(s), under exclusive license to Springer Nature 105
Switzerland AG 2025
L. Sera, C. Hempel-Sanderoff, *Cannabis Science and Therapeutics*,
https://doi.org/10.1007/978-3-031-80352-9_8

contain up to 80–90% THC [2]. The risks of consuming high-potency cannabis products are becoming increasingly clear, with increased risk of addiction and rising reports of conditions such as cannabis hyperemesis syndrome, first-episode psychosis, and emergency department encounters for cannabis toxicity [3–7]. Any approach to counseling patients about medical cannabis should include a clear warning about the dangers associated with using high-potency cannabis products and a recommendation to avoid them.

8.2   In the Weeds: Practical Matters Related to Managing Cannabis-Based Medicine

The tables and discussion in this chapter are intended to provide the clinician with a quick reference for important information related to common cannabis formulations, dosing strategies, and important variables to consider when managing cannabis-based medicines (Tables 8.1, 8.2, 8.3 and 8.4).

Table 8.1 Characteristics of inhaled cannabis product formulations

Formulation	Onset/duration [15]	Advantages	Disadvantages
Dried cannabis flower	Onset: 5–10 min Duration: 2–4 h	• Dried flower is activated using combustion or vaporized using heated coils • Quickly enters bloodstream and CNS for rapid onset • Helpful for quick symptom relief	• Smoke and combustion byproducts can be irritating • Difficult to dose and titrate due to individual inhalation techniques • Unclear risks to lung health[a]

(continued)

Table 8.1 (continued)

Formulation	Onset/duration [15]	Advantages	Disadvantages
Cannabis oil	Onset: 5–10 min Duration: 2–4 h	Not recommended for medical use	• Oil extracted from cannabis plants is heated and inhaled using a battery-powered device or cartridge, also known as vaping • Can be highly concentrated with unpredictable effects • Oils can contain additives or contaminants • Recent outbreak of lung disease from contaminated vape cartridges (VALI) [8]
Cannabis concentrates Numerous names: • Wax • Shatter • Batter • Budder • Sugar	Onset: 5–10 min Duration: Unpredictable but usually 2–4 h	Not recommended for medical use	• Highly concentrated extracts of THC (40–80%), usually chemically extracted • Must be heated using high heat and a blowtorch apparatus

[a]Vaporized cannabis flower is heated using coils and not combustion, considered to be less irritating than smoking

Table 8.2 Characteristics of buccal or oromucosal products

Formulation	Onset/ duration [15]	Advantages	Disadvantages
Tinctures[a]	Onset: 15–45 min Duration: 6–8 h	• Simple to select desired dose • Drops administered under the tongue • Easier to give small doses • Fairly predictable effects • Recommended for patients new to medical cannabis	• May be difficult for patients with dexterity or vision issues • May contain additives
Lozenges or troches	Onset: 15–45 min Duration: 6–8 h	• Simple to select desired dose • Dissolves under the tongue • Recommended for patients new to medical cannabis	• May contain additives, sugars, and flavorings
Sprays	Onset: 15–45 min Duration: 6–8 h	• Simple to select desired dose and titrate in small amounts • Spray dose directly under tongue	• May be difficult for patients with dexterity issues • Pharmaceutical preparation not widely available in the United States

[a]Tinctures may have similar onset to oral products when swallowed

Table 8.3 Characteristics of oral products

Formulation	Onset/duration [15]	Advantages	Disadvantages
Capsules or tablets	Onset: 1–3 h Duration: Unpredictable but typically 6–8 h	• Simple to select desired dose • More discreet • May provide longer-lasting therapeutic effect	• Poor bioavailability • Effects can be unpredictable • Adverse effects are also long-lasting • Challenging to titrate

(continued)

Table 8.3 (continued)

Formulation	Onset/duration [15]	Advantages	Disadvantages
Gummies	Onset: 1–3 h Duration: 6–8 h	• Simple to select desired dose • Discreet • Generally palatable, flavored	• Poor bioavailability • Unpredictable effects that can be long-lasting • Watch for additives, flavorings, and sugar content

Table 8.4 Characteristics of topical and transdermal products

Formulation	Onset/duration [15]	Advantages	Disadvantages
Topical[a]	Limited data	• Little to no systemic absorption • Non-impairing • May be helpful for localized pain	• Variable absorption • Variable cannabinoid content
Transdermal	Onset: 1–7 h Duration: Up to 24–72 h	• Absorbed systemically into the bloodstream • Long duration	• May be impairing • Highly variable absorption • Unpredictable effects • Challenging to dose • Not widely available

[a]Topical products frequently contain other topical pain relievers

8.3   An Individualized Approach to Dosing and Titration

Each patient should be approached with an understanding of their unique conditions, symptoms, and goals. In Chap. 9, you can review sample patient encounters with examples of how to apply these considerations. Here are the key areas for clinicians to include in an evaluation or when counseling patients regarding medical cannabis therapies.

8.3.1   Cannabis Use History

Ask patients if they have any prior experience with cannabis. It is very helpful to understand previous cannabis use patterns and their effects. Some patients are currently using cannabis or have used cannabis in the past but have not previously discussed it with a healthcare professional. Asking about their experiences can provide insight into their unique ECS function. If a patient reports pleasant experiences versus unpleasant effects, paranoia, or cognitive impairment with past use, this can aid in anticipating the potential effects of cannabis for their current symptoms. For example, patients with prior negative experiences using cannabis should be directed toward CBD-dominant formulations to minimize the risk of adverse effects of THC. Creating an environment that favors candid discussion is essential for overcoming stigma. Discussions with patients about prior cannabis use should be non-judgmental and supportive to facilitate openness and communication.

8.3.2   Patient-Related Variables

While there are few absolute contraindications to medical cannabis use, the presence of coexisting conditions can increase risk and warrant closer monitoring. Cannabis use can worsen cardiac arrhythmias, hypotension, and cardiovascular disease [9]. Mental health conditions such as anxiety, depression, bipolar disorder, and PTSD may also worsen with the initiation of cannabis (particularly THC-containing formulations) [4]. Patients with visual impairment or dexterity issues may struggle to dose and administer liquid tinctures or to read labels, and patients with congestive obstructive pulmonary disease (COPD) or respiratory issues will need to avoid smoking or inhaled formulations. These coexisting conditions must be explored with patients to optimize the informed selection of an ideal formulation.

8.3.3   Formulation Preference

Another step in creating an individualized approach to medical cannabis is to understand the general categories of cannabis for-

Table 8.5 Cannabinoid ratios [10]

Cannabis type	Characteristics
Type I • High THC/CBD ratio • THC-dominant	• Most impairing • Highest proportion of THC • Most popular with social or recreational cannabis users • Less medical usefulness
Type II • Balanced CBD/THC ratio • Equal cannabinoid proportions	• May be impairing • Better for severe symptoms or prior cannabis experience • Use more caution with titration
Type III • High CBD/THC ratio • CBD-dominant	• Low impairment risk • Ideal for initiation or cannabis-naive patients • Usually well-tolerated

mulations and CBD/THC ratios that are available to patients in your state (see Table 8.5 for types and characteristics of cannabis products). After discussing the pros and cons of the different formulations, patients may have certain preferences for how they wish to consume cannabis. Inhaled forms of cannabis are not considered first-line therapies. However, an example of when this might be considered is a patient with terminal cancer who is unable to swallow pills or food. They may only be able to achieve pain and nausea relief by inhaling (i.e., smoking or vaporizing) cannabis. In this situation, the patient's preference for an inhaled formulation is reasonable and could be supported, given the situation and goals. Some patients with children at home prefer more discreet formulations without odor that can be locked and stored safely away. Other patients may not want to ingest cannabis at all and prefer to try topical formulations. Having a broad understanding of the availability of products in your state can significantly aid discussions about potential medical cannabis treatment options.

8.4 Dosing Strategies

Aside from the few FDA-approved cannabis-based medicines for chemotherapy-induced nausea and vomiting and pediatric seizure disorders (refer to Table 3.2 for a list of available cannabinoid preparations), there are currently no disease-specific approaches to medical cannabis dosing. Since the general properties and effects of the ECS are scientifically understood, several panels of international experts have recently developed a guided approach to initiation, titration, and monitoring for medicinal doses of cannabis [11]. The mantra remains: "Start low and go slow." In this section, we will describe some dosing recommendations for cannabis-naive patients and patients with cannabis experience or severe symptoms. It is essential to approach all prospective patients interested in using medical cannabis on an individual basis, considering their unique characteristics and goals. Please note that these dosing recommendations are limited to oral and oromucosal formulations. The high variability of cannabinoid content, the individual inhalation techniques, and the potential risks of smoking cannabis are prohibitive to the creation of standardized dosing or clinical recommendations for inhaled cannabis.

8.4.1   A Conservative Approach for Cannabis-Naïve Patients

Although the thought of using cannabis as medicine may conjure up a mental image of long hair, bell-bottom jeans, and the Grateful Dead, the reality is that many patients interested in medical cannabis have never used it before. Often, the stigma and taboo nature of messaging around cannabis over the past century has influenced patients' perceptions and openness to exploring cannabis medicine. With rapidly expanding access and numerous anecdotal reports of symptom relief, patients are now overcoming this hesitancy. A conservative approach, using low doses of CBD and THC, is recommended for cannabis-naïve patients, which reduces the risk of unwanted impairment. This approach may also be used for patients who have experience with cannabis; for these patients, larger doses of THC (2.5 mg compared to 1 mg) can be used during titration if THC is needed for symptom management. Patients with cannabis experience may be able to tolerate higher doses of THC without adverse effects.

8.4.2 Rapid Titration for Patients with Severe Symptoms

Patients with severe symptoms or who have tolerance to the effects of cannabis may require higher doses of THC to achieve therapeutic effects and also tend to tolerate such doses without significant impairment. A rapid titration approach is described in Tables 8.6 and 8.7.

Table 8.6 Sample conservative dosing approach with type III cannabis (CBD-dominant) [11]

		Suggested dosing		Titration strategy
Initial dose	⟶	5 mg CBD once or twice daily	⟶	Increase CBD dose by 10 mg every 2–3 days until relief is felt
If no relief is felt after 40 mg CBD daily	⟶	Add 1–2.5 mg THC daily	⟶	Increase THC dose by 1 mg daily every 7 days
If no relief after 40 mg THC daily or presence of adverse effects	⟶	Consider stopping treatment		

Table 8.7 Sample rapid titration approach with type II cannabis (balanced THC/CBD) [11]

		Suggested dosing		Titration strategy
Initial dose	⟶	2.5 mg of each (CBD and THC) once or twice daily	⟶	Increase both doses by 2.5 mg once or twice daily every 2–3 days
If no relief after 40 mg THC daily or presence of adverse effects	⟶	Consider stopping treatment		

8.5   Approach to Monitoring

Monitoring for efficacy (i.e., symptom improvement) and toxicity (i.e., adverse effects) is essential during the first weeks of medical cannabis initiation and titration. Many patients tolerate low doses of THC and CBD without significant impairment; however, in some cases where patients are very sensitive to THC psychoactivity, unpleasant side effects can occur. The most common adverse effects include dry mouth, dizziness, sedation, and cognitive impairment [12]. Higher doses of THC cause worsening impairment, along with other adverse effects such as visual changes, hypotension, gait disturbance, tachycardia, paranoia, psychosis, or GI effects, including nausea, vomiting, and diarrhea [12]. In clinical trials, CBD has been associated with somnolence, fatigue, and GI upset. High doses of CBD may be associated with increased liver function transaminase levels [13].

Patients using medical cannabis concomitantly with other medications may be at risk for pharmacokinetic or pharmacodynamic drug-drug interactions. Pharmacokinetic drug interactions occur because one drug reduces or induces the metabolism of another, typically via modulation of CYP enzymes in the liver. This can lead to supratherapeutic drug levels, on the one hand, with the potential for increased toxicity, or subtherapeutic drug levels, on the other hand, with a risk of decreased effectiveness. Pharmacodynamic drug interactions occur because one drug's pharmacologic effects modulate another's pharmacologic effects. Table 8.8 describes selected clinically relevant drug-drug interactions. This is not an exhaustive list, so keep in mind the hypothetical risk for interactions with drugs that are affected by hepatic metabolism; this is an especially important consideration for patients experiencing polypharmacy (many medications).

Based on the suggested dosing and titration schedules above, the ideal follow-up window is during the first 1–2 weeks of starting medical cannabis. Once dosing and frequency are stable and assuming the patient does not experience adverse effects, the follow-up interval can be increased to monthly or bi-monthly. Clinicians should tailor their treatment plans to individual patients,

Table 8.8 Selected clinically relevant cannabinoid drug-drug interactions [14]

Drug class Drug(s)	Interacts with THC	CBD	Interaction type PK	PD	Comments
Anticoagulants Warfarin	x	x	x		• May increase warfarin concentration • Monitor for evidence of warfarin toxicity (e.g., bleeding) • Consider cannabinoid dose reduction
Antidepressants Citalopram		x	x	x	• May increase citalopram concentration • Risk of additive sedation and cognitive impairment • Monitor for evidence of citalopram toxicity (e.g., serotonin syndrome)
Benzodiazepines Clobazam		x	x		• May increase clobazam concentration • Monitor therapy and consider reduction in clobazam dose
CNS depressants	x	x		x	• Monitor therapy • Consider reduction of cannabinoid dose
Anticholinergics	x			x	• May enhance the tachycardic effect of THC • Consider reduction of cannabinoid dose

PK pharmacokinetic, *PD* pharmacodynamic

their conditions, and their needs. Patients are often encouraged to keep a symptom log or journal to track their doses and responses to treatment to assist with this process.

Red flags or indications to consider discontinuing medical cannabis include daily THC dosing greater than 40 mg without symptom relief or with worsening symptoms or adverse effects. Positive responses when screening for dependence, seeking behavior, or other concerns for CUD should also prompt counseling or consideration of alternate therapies.

References

1. ElSohly MA, Mehmedic Z, Foster S, Gon C, Chandra S, Church JC. Changes in cannabis potency over the last 2 decades (1995–2014): analysis of current data in the United States. Biol Psychiatry. 2016;79(7):613–9. https://doi.org/10.1016/j.biopsych.2016.01.004. Epub 2016 Jan 19. PMID: 26903403; PMCID: PMC4987131.
2. Drug Enforcement Administration. Facts about marijuana concentrates [Internet]. https://www.justthinktwice.gov/facts-about-marijuana-concentrates. Accessed 2 Sep 2024.
3. Connor JP, Stjepanović D, Le Foll B, Hoch E, Budney AJ, Hall WD. Cannabis use and cannabis use disorder. Nat Rev Dis Primers. 2021;7(1):16. https://doi.org/10.1038/s41572-021-00247-4. PMID: 33627670; PMCID: PMC8655458.
4. Petrilli K, Ofori S, Hines L, Taylor G, Adams S, Freeman TP. Association of cannabis potency with mental ill health and addiction: a systematic review. Lancet Psychiatry. 2022;9(9):736–50. https://doi.org/10.1016/S2215-0366(22)00161-4. Epub 2022 Jul 25.
5. Schoeler T, Ferris J, Winstock AR. Rates and correlates of cannabis-associated psychotic symptoms in over 230,000 people who use cannabis. Transl Psychiatry. 2022;12(1):369. https://doi.org/10.1038/s41398-022-02112-8. PMID: 36068202; PMCID: PMC9448725.
6. Di Forti M, Marconi A, Carra E, Fraietta S, Trotta A, Bonomo M, Bianconi F, Gardner-Sood P, O'Connor J, Russo M, Stilo SA, Marques TR, Mondelli V, Dazzan P, Pariante C, David AS, Gaughran F, Atakan Z, Iyegbe C, Powell J, Morgan C, Lynskey M, Murray RM. Proportion of patients in South London with first-episode psychosis attributable to use of high potency cannabis: a case-control study. Lancet Psychiatry. 2015;2(3):233–8. https://doi.org/10.1016/S2215-0366(14)00117-5. Epub 2015 Feb 25.
7. Senderovich H, Patel P, Jimenez Lopez B, Waicus S. A systematic review on cannabis hyperemesis syndrome and its management options. Med Princ Pract. 2022;31(1):29–38. https://doi.org/10.1159/000520417. Epub 2021 Nov 1. PMID: 34724666; PMCID: PMC8995641.
8. Adapa S, Gayam V, Konala VM, Annangi S, Raju MP, Bezwada V, McMillan C, Dalal H, Mandal A, Naramala S. Cannabis vaping-induced acute pulmonary toxicity: case series and review of literature. J Investig Med High Impact Case Rep. 2020;8:2324709620947267. https://doi.org/10.1177/2324709620947267. PMID: 32755249; PMCID: PMC7543135.
9. Jeffers AM, Glantz S, Byers AL, Keyhani S. Association of cannabis use with cardiovascular outcomes among US adults. J Am Heart Assoc. 2024;13(5):e030178. https://doi.org/10.1161/JAHA.123.030178. Epub 2024 Feb 28. PMID: 38415581; PMCID: PMC10944074.

10. Blesching U. The cannabis health index: combining the science of medical marijuana with mindfulness techniques to treat over 200 chronic diseases. 3rd ed. Berkeley, California: Logos/Uwe Blesching; 2022.
11. Bhaskar A, Bell A, Boivin M, Briques W, Brown M, Clarke H, Cyr C, Eisenberg E, de Oliveira Silva RF, Frohlich E, Georgius P, Hogg M, Horsted TI, MacCallum CA, Müller-Vahl KR, O'Connell C, Sealey R, Seibolt M, Sihota A, Smith BK, Sulak D, Vigano A, Moulin DE. Consensus recommendations on dosing and administration of medical cannabis to treat chronic pain: results of a modified Delphi process. J Cannabis Res. 2021;3(1):22. https://doi.org/10.1186/s42238-021-00073-1. PMID: 34215346; PMCID: PMC8252988.
12. Urits I, Charipova K, Gress K, Li N, Berger AA, Cornett EM, Kassem H, Ngo AL, Kaye AD, Viswanath O. Adverse effects of recreational and medical cannabis. Psychopharmacol Bull. 2021;51(1):94–109. PMID: 33897066; PMCID: PMC8063125.
13. Huestis MA, Solimini R, Pichini S, Pacifici R, Carlier J, Busardò FP. Cannabidiol adverse effects and toxicity. Curr Neuropharmacol. 2019;17(10):974–89. https://doi.org/10.2174/15701 59X17666190603171901. PMID: 31161980; PMCID: PMC7052834.
14. Sera L, Duncan N. Medical cannabis: roles, responsibilities, and challenges for clinical pharmacists. JAACP. 2023;6(7):732–41.
15. MacCallum CA, Russo EB. Practical considerations in medical cannabis administration and dosing. Eur J Int Med. 2018;49:12–9.

In this final chapter, the information in the book is combined with adapted real-world clinical case examples. This practical illustration of the unique individual approaches and considerations seeks to provide readily applicable guidance for counseling and supporting patients in the evolving era of medical cannabis.

9.1 Case No. 1: Anxiety

9.1.1 Background/Chief Complaint

Mary is a 56-year-old woman who comes to your office asking if cannabis will help with her anxiety. Recently, she was talking to a friend who reported using cannabis gummies from the dispensary with good effects. Mary is now wondering if she should try them for the management of daily anxiety, hypervigilance, and occasional panic attacks.

9.1.2 History of Present Illness

Mary reports having anxious feelings for most of her adult life. She can't isolate a specific event that precipitated her chronic anxiety; she describes it as a daily feeling of discomfort, hyper-

© The Author(s), under exclusive license to Springer Nature Switzerland AG 2025
L. Sera, C. Hempel-Sanderoff, *Cannabis Science and Therapeutics*, https://doi.org/10.1007/978-3-031-80352-9_9

vigilance, and situational fearfulness. She received a diagnosis of generalized anxiety disorder from her primary care provider (PCP) 10 years ago and has tried several traditional pharmaceutical medications with partial improvement. She still has daily symptoms and occasional panic attacks about once per month.

9.1.3   Medical, Surgical, and Social History

Aside from this, she is relatively healthy, with a prior history of hypothyroidism, hyperlipidemia, and vitamin D deficiency. She denies a personal or family history of psychosis, schizophrenia, or substance abuse disorders. She is semi-retired and works part-time at a community center as an event organizer. She is married and has two grown children who live out of town.

9.1.4   Current Medications

- Escitalopram 20 mg daily—taking for 2 years.
- Levothyroxine 75 μg daily—taking for 10 years, recent thyroid studies stable.
- Atorvastatin 40 mg daily—taking for 10 years, no issues, LFTs normal.
- ASA 81 mg—daily for "heart protection".
- Alprazolam 0.25 mg as needed—taking 2–3 times per month for severe symptoms or panic attacks.

9.1.5   Cannabis Use History and Preferences

Mary tried smoking cannabis in her late teens and early 20 s during college but didn't like the effects, stating it made her feel anxious and paranoid. She does not smoke cigarettes or drink alcohol. She does not want to smoke or use any inhaled cannabis products. Her preference is an oral formula or tincture for discreet use and storage. She does not want to feel any impairment or use THC, which she fears would make her symptoms worse.

9.1.6   Assessment

Mary is a good candidate for medical cannabis. Based on her history and prior cannabis experience, the best choice of cannabinoid ratio is type III, with little or no THC and predominant CBD. Literature review suggests that CBD is the cannabinoid with the most evidence for benefit in chronic and situational anxiety [1].

9.1.7   Recommendation

Based on CBD dosages in studies and recent expert consensus guidelines, a starting dosage of 5 mg CBD twice daily is recommended.

9.1.8   Treatment Course, Counseling, and Monitoring

- Based on her medication history, Mary is at moderate risk for drug-drug interactions. Potential additive sedation is possible when paired with alprazolam, so she is advised to use caution or avoid taking them together.

- Mary is advised to keep a symptom journal to track her progress and responses.
- The first follow-up visit should be scheduled within 1–2 weeks to assess her response and titrate dosage if needed. Follow up every 1–2 weeks until the dose and symptoms are stabilized. Subsequent follow-up is based on Mary's needs and should occur at least every 6 months.
- Mary returns 2 weeks later and reports minimal effects from her starting dosage. Over the next 2 weeks, she slowly increases her daily dose to 20 mg twice daily.
- When she returns for her 1-month follow-up, she reports feeling noticeably calmer and more relaxed. She is happy to report that she has had no panic attacks and needed no alprazolam in the past month. She denies adverse effects, GI symptoms, somnolence, or other negative effects.
- Two months later, Mary returns and reports feeling much calmer and more at ease. She did have one panic attack 3 weeks ago, for which she used alprazolam, but these occurrences are significantly reduced. No drug interactions are suspected, and her primary care physician (PCP) will monitor her thyroid and liver function twice yearly.
- One year later, Mary continues to do well using CBD 20 mg twice daily as an adjunct to her escitalopram. She has an occasional panic attack every 2–3 months, but she reports that they are much less intense, and she can breathe through them rather than taking alprazolam. For now, her escitalopram dose is unchanged, but she plans to ask her PCP about the possibility of reducing it if her anxiety continues to improve.

9.2   Case No. 2: Insomnia

9.2.1   Background/Chief Complaint

John is a 49-year-old man who comes to see you for a medical cannabis consultation. He wonders if he needs something "stronger" to help him sleep.

9.2.2   History of Present Illness

John has a history of shift work, including night shifts, over the past 15 years. He likes to relax by going to the casino or the race-track, sometimes losing more money than he can spare and stay-ing up all night. His sleep schedule is erratic and inconsistent from week to week. He hasn't seen a primary care doctor for at least 5 years. When asked about his treatment goals, he can only state, "I just want to be able to sleep when I need to."

9.2.3   Medical, Surgical, and Social History

John has some health issues, including hypertension, high choles-terol, and chronic kidney disease. The patient and his family mem-bers often report that he is "moody" and can become withdrawn and irritable, especially with a lack of sleep. He has been a cigarette smoker for 20 years, and he drinks 4–6 beers daily. He is divorced and has two children, ages 8 and 12, with shared custody. His aging mother lives with him and assists with childcare. The family is frag-mented with poor social support, and he has two siblings who are estranged due to emotional outbursts and aggression. His father died by suicide when John was a teenager. John uses alcohol and tobacco daily and uses cannabis several times a week (see below).

9.2.4   Current Medications

He is prescribed medications for his blood pressure and choles-terol but chooses not to take them.

9.2.5   Cannabis Use History and Preferences

John reports smoking cannabis 3–4 times per week. He has "smoked weed" off and on for most of his adult life, but recently, it has been making him paranoid and restless.

Questions for the Clinician

Before reading further, pause to consider the following questions:

1. Is John's insomnia currently well controlled?
2. What first- and/or second-line treatments has John tried, and how effective have they been?
3. Does John have any contraindications to cannabis treatment or precautions to consider?
4. If you decide to recommend medical cannabis for John, what formulation/product is appropriate?
5. Does John require any special monitoring based on his medical or medication history?

9.2.6   Assessment

This case requires a cautious and discerning approach. In John's history, there are several red flags suggesting a higher risk for adverse outcomes. His current substance use and gambling patterns are concerning for a tendency toward addictive behaviors. Also, his mood and irritability, along with his family history, raise concerns about mental health conditions. Additionally, he has a history of poor adherence to other treatment recommendations and prescription medications. John is already using cannabis several times per week with no improvement in sleep. These factors make John a poor candidate for medical cannabis treatment.

The current evidence for cannabis-based treatment of insomnia remains scant and conflicting. Although cannabis is known for its relaxing and sedating effects, and the ECS appears to help regulate sleep cycles, the true effects remain unknown. One systematic review indicated benefits from THC and CBD on sleep onset and REM sleep, but there are still no definitive RCTs to provide clinicians with robust, high-quality evidence to aid in decision-making [2].

9.2.7   Recommendations

John is a poor candidate for medical cannabis treatment, and it should not be recommended for him at this time. His history of poor adherence to treatment plans will make it challenging to provide dosing and formulation guidance and reliably monitor his responses. An ideal plan for John would be a compassionate discussion about the risks of his lifestyle and substance use, with a referral back to his primary care doctor for follow-up and additional evaluation.

9.3   Case No. 3: Post-Traumatic Stress Disorder (PTSD)

9.3.1   Background/Chief Complaint

Bill is a 62-year-old combat veteran who served in the Vietnam War. When he returned from the war in the late 1970s, he struggled to reassimilate into society. He has a formal diagnosis of PTSD, and he attends treatment groups and therapy sessions occasionally but has resisted pharmaceutical treatment due to his fear of being poisoned. He is hoping that medical cannabis can help with his PTSD symptoms.

9.3.2   History of Present Illness

When Bill returned from the war in the 1970s, he struggled to reassimilate into society. He was unable to maintain steady employment and became homeless for several years. He was then hospitalized for almost a year after being hit by a car, during which time he was formally diagnosed with PTSD. After that hospitalization, he entered a VA physical rehabilitation program and received stable residential care. After he recovered, he moved to a small apartment and lived on a stipend. He has intermittent part-time work but continues to struggle with employment due to his unpredictable moods, out-of-proportion reactions, and erratic behavior. Loud and crowded work environments are intolerable to him.

9.3.3   Medical, Surgical, and Social History

In addition to PTSD, Bill has a history of hypertension (currently controlled without medication use), congestive obstructive pulmonary disorder (COPD), and paroxysmal atrial fibrillation. He suffered a fracture of the left femur 20 years ago. Bill smokes one half to one pack per day to "calm his nerves." He doesn't drink because "alcohol tastes like poison." He lives alone but has a community of veterans for support and socializing when he feels well enough. His parents and brother are deceased, and he has minimal contact with other family members.

9.3.4   Current Medications

- Aspirin 81 mg daily.
- Albuterol inhaler as needed.

9.3.5   Cannabis Use History and Preferences

One of Bill's friends smokes cannabis regularly and Bill has been joining him 2–3 times per month for the past year. After smoking a small amount of cannabis, Bill feels more relaxed and even calm. He can laugh and participate in conversations and "sleeps like a baby" that night. He feels calmer for a few days after that, but eventually, his symptoms return until the next time he smokes cannabis. One time, after smoking a little too much, he started to feel more anxious and paranoid, so now he limits himself to 2–3 puffs in each session.

Questions for the Clinician

Before reading further, pause to consider the following questions:

1. Is Bill's PTSD currently well controlled?
2. What first- and/or second-line treatments has Bill tried, and how effective have they been?
3. Does Bill have any contraindications to cannabis treatment or precautions to consider?
4. If you decide to recommend medical cannabis for Bill, what formulation/product is appropriate?
5. Does Bill require any special monitoring based on his medical or medication history?

9.3.6 Assessment

Bill's PTSD has affected his life profoundly. Although his interpersonal challenges have limited him, and his employment has been erratic, he has experienced symptomatic relief and improved quality of life with cannabis use. Bill has some risks due to his coexisting conditions, specifically his COPD and atrial fibrillation. Smoking cannabis can cause bronchial inflammation, worsen lung function, and increase cancer risk [3]. THC can also increase the risk of cardiac arrhythmia [4]. He is somewhat resistant to medications but will take aspirin and uses an albuterol inhaler occasionally. These have minimal risk of interaction with cannabis. However, untreated cardiovascular conditions can be exacerbated by cannabis, again warranting caution.

Bill has smoked one pack of cigarettes daily for about 40 years, and he does have COPD. He does not drink alcohol or use other substances, and he reports avoiding high doses of cannabis, self-monitoring his degree of impairment, and moderating his intake, which is less concerning for his risk of addiction. His familial mental health history is unknown, and his current mental health condition warrants close monitoring if he is using cannabis.

Given the severity of Bill's symptoms, their impact on his quality of life, and his resistance to medication management of his PTSD, he would be a candidate for a trial of medical cannabis for his PTSD symptoms. Given his higher risks, regular follow-up and close monitoring will be necessary.

9.3.7   Recommendations

Bill should avoid smoking cannabis. Although this is a commonly used and widely available formulation, Bill's lung health is already at risk due to his tobacco use and COPD diagnosis, and part of Bill's visit should include counseling about this risk, with a recommendation to use other formulations. Bill agrees to try cannabis gummies that he will obtain at the local dispensary. He asks if they are safe, how long they will last, and how well they will work. Since Bill is an experienced cannabis user, he could follow a more rapid dosing and titration protocol (see Table 8.7). The recommended dose is 2.5 mg CBD/2.5 mg THC twice daily. Since many gummy products are sold in doses of 5 or 10 mg per gummy, this dose would be one half gummy twice daily.

Example Language for Counseling Bill
- "Bill, I am glad to hear that smoking cannabis has given you symptom relief and made you feel more comfortable. There is currently no definitive proof that cannabis helps PTSD, but patients just like you are reporting positive effects. Because of your COPD and cigarette smoking, I'm worried that smoking cannabis will make your lungs worse. It's not the safest way for you to get symptom relief with cannabis. I recommend a different type of cannabis product, administered under the tongue or by mouth, that could give you similar relief without causing more lung damage. Would you be willing to try treatment with a liquid, tablet, or edible cannabis formulation?"

- "To keep track of how your body responds to each dose of the cannabis gummy, use a small journal or notepad to record how your symptoms change after using the product and how long the effects last. In general, cannabis products that you eat or take by mouth take 1–2 h to take effect, so be careful not to re-dose if you don't feel anything right away. If the dose is right for you, you should feel relaxed but not impaired. This effect generally lasts 4–6 h, but it can differ for everyone. When we see each other again, we can discuss your results and decide together if adjustments are needed."

9.3.8   Treatment Course, Counseling, and Monitoring

- Bill purchases cannabis gummies from the dispensary containing 5 mg CBD and 5 mg THC (1:1 ratio, type II formulation).
- At the 1-week follow-up visit, he reports minimal improvement and no noticeable adverse effects.
- Given this, the dose is increased to one gummy (5 mg CBD/5 mg THC twice daily).
- At the next 1-week follow-up visit, he reports feeling more relaxed through the day, and he noticed that he is falling asleep after 30 min at night rather than tossing and turning for 2–3 h. He doesn't feel "stoned" or impaired. He sleeps well and wakes up feeling rested, with no residual grogginess.
- Bill is happy with these results so far. He doesn't like to feel impaired or out of control, and he is pleasantly surprised at the more gradual and longer-lasting effects of the gummies. He will continue to avoid or minimize smoking cannabis since these products are helping his symptoms.
- Additional follow-up continues at 2-month intervals until dose and symptoms are stable and then at 6-month intervals as Bill's dosage and products remain stable. He has not demonstrated CUD behaviors and is avoiding high-potency cannabis. He reports continued improvement in his quality of life and his comfort levels.

9.4   Case No. 4: Chronic Pain

9.4.1   Background/Chief Complaint

Nancy is a 62-year-old female with longstanding chronic pain from osteoarthritis and diabetic neuropathy. She is interested in exploring medical cannabis as an adjunct to current pain management therapies.

9.4.2   History of Present Illness

Nancy likes to be active and enjoys walking her dog and playing with her grandchildren. Over the past 15 years, she has developed arthritis in both knees, along with diabetes and associated neuropathy. Over the past 3 years, her knee and leg pain have become much more bothersome. She reports daily feelings of numbness and tingling in her feet that now keeps her awake at night. Her knees have become swollen, and she can't tolerate walking long distances or excessive movement. Her primary care doctor prescribed gabapentin for her neuropathic pain, and she has been using acetaminophen and a topical pain relief cream on her knees.

Nancy is not ready for knee replacement surgery yet, and she does not want to try stronger pain medications. She hopes to reduce her pain enough to be able to go on walks with her husband and her dog and to reduce her neuropathic pain at night. She reports that most days, her knee and leg pain are 7/10. She acknowledges that she is unlikely to reach a pain-free state, but she feels that she could function more comfortably at a pain level of 3/10.

9.4.3   Medical, Surgical, and Social History

Nancy has a past medical history of hypertension, type II diabetes, and osteoarthritis. She is a retired schoolteacher. She lives with her husband of 35 years. They have one grown son and two grandchildren who visit often. Nancy has never smoked and drinks alcohol rarely, less than once per month.

9.4.4   Current Medications

- Lisinopril 5 mg daily for hypertension.
- Metformin 1000 mg twice daily for diabetes.
- Sitagliptin 100 mg daily for diabetes.
- Gabapentin 400 mg twice daily for neuropathic pain.
- Acetaminophen 1000 mg three times daily.

9.4.5   Cannabis Use History and Preferences

Nancy has never used cannabis before.

Questions for the Clinician

Before reading further, pause to consider the following questions:

1. Are Nancy's arthritis and neuropathy currently well controlled?
2. What first- and/or second-line treatments has Nancy tried, and how effective have they been?
3. Does Nancy have any contraindications to cannabis treatment or precautions to consider?
4. If you decide to recommend medical cannabis for Nancy, what formulation/product is appropriate?
5. Does Nancy require any special monitoring based on her medical or medication history?

9.4.6   Assessment

Nancy is a good candidate for a trial of medical cannabis for her multifactorial chronic pain. The two symptoms she is hoping to treat are neuropathic pain and chronic inflammatory knee pain. Medical cannabis appears to help reduce both types of pain in numerous studies (though the overall strength of evidence is low as most studies are small with varying methodologies), and patients do report measurable pain reduction with both THC and CBD [5–7]. Nancy's conditions are progressing despite standard treatments, making a trial of cannabis-based medicine reasonable.

9.4.7   Recommendations

Since Nancy is cannabis-naive, her ideal starting cannabis formulation would be a type III cannabis formulation that is high in CBD, with little or no THC. Nancy prefers to be cautious and does not want to feel high or impaired, so she chooses to start with CBD only (no THC). The recommended starting dose is CBD 5 mg twice daily.

9.4.8   Treatment Course, Counseling, and Monitoring

- CBD may interact with gabapentin, resulting in additive sedation. Counsel Nancy to watch for this while taking CBD, and her gabapentin dose might need to be decreased if this happens.
- For the first 7 days, Nancy notices no significant effects. At her 1-week follow-up visit, the dose is increased to 10 mg twice daily. She still reports no improvement or effects. Over the next 3 weeks, the dose is titrated until Nancy is taking 20 mg twice daily.
- At her 1-month follow-up visit, she is beginning to feel some improvement. Her knee pain has decreased from 7/10 to 5/10, but her nighttime neuropathic pain is still unchanged. Since

she is not experiencing negative side effects or sedation, she is open to adding THC to her regimen.

- Her local dispensary carries a tincture with a 10:1 ratio of CBD/THC (10 mg CBD and 1 mg THC per 1 mL dropper). She switches to this formula and begins to take one dropperful twice daily.

- At her next visit, she reports being surprised and happy with the addition of a small dose of THC. Her pain levels have decreased to 2/10, and her neuropathic pain has improved enough that she is sleeping more comfortably. She is using acetaminophen only twice per day now rather than three times per day.

- After 2 more weeks, she feels confident and encouraged by her progress and jokes about her new "hippie lifestyle." Over the next 6–12 months, she continues to integrate medical cannabis into her care as you follow with her.

9.5   Case No. 5: Cancer and Cancer Symptoms

9.5.1   Background/Chief Complaint

Mike is a 66-year-old male with stage IV colon cancer. He wants to know if medical cannabis can improve his symptoms and quality of life.

9.5.2   History of Present Illness

Four years ago, Mike noticed a change in his stools and more difficulty having bowel movements. Two years ago, when he began to see blood in his stool, he saw a GI specialist who performed a colonoscopy and found a large mass in his sigmoid colon. A biopsy confirmed adenocarcinoma of the colon. He was found to have metastasis to his pelvic lymph nodes and two liver masses also suspicious for metastasis. Further imaging confirmed metastasis to the liver along with two spinal metastases.

Over the following 2 years, Mike's cancer was treated with surgery to remove the sigmoid mass and improve bowel function, creating a colostomy and hepatic embolization of his liver lesions. He is now taking capecitabine and pembrolizumab with the continued hope of slowing disease progression and optimizing his life span.

Mike's diagnosis of stage IV colon cancer and the subsequent surgery, chemotherapies, and cancer progression have been challenging for him. In the past 2 years, he has lost 50 pounds and struggles with daily nausea, poor appetite, abdominal pain, and diarrhea. His bone metastases are becoming very painful. He refuses to use opioid pain medications due to "not wanting to be addicted" but is open to considering other treatment options to feel better. His goal is to "feel as good as I can" and to "be around as long as I can" to spend quality time with his family and grandchildren.

9.5.3   Medical, Surgical, and Social History

In addition to colon cancer, Mike has a past medical history of hypertension and hyperlipidemia. Before his colon cancer diagnosis, Mike was in good health. He has owned a plumbing business for 30 years and works long hours managing his employees and running a busy and successful plumbing business. He has been married to his wife for almost 40 years. They live together in a large family home with his elderly mother-in-law, who is debilitated and requires care. They have two grown adult children who live locally and three grandchildren who are toddlers.

Mike has smoked cigarettes for most of his adult life, although he has now quit smoking due to his cancer diagnosis. He enjoys drinking beer after work and on the weekends to relax and will consume 2–6 beers in a sitting.

9.5.4   Current Medications

- Amlodipine 5 mg daily for hypertension.
- Atorvastatin 10 mg daily for hyperlipidemia.

9.5.5 Cannabis Use History and Preferences

Mike reports smoking cannabis "years ago" in his 20 s and remembers feeling happy and finding it socially enjoyable. He has not used cannabis since then. Mike doesn't want to smoke due to the odor and is concerned about vomiting while coughing. He has trouble keeping pills down but could tolerate a buccal or oromucosal formulation. He doesn't like the idea of a tincture due to concerns about vomiting, but he is interested in a lozenge or troche that would dissolve in his mouth.

Questions for the Clinician
Before reading further, pause to consider the following questions:

1. Are the symptoms resulting from Mike's cancer and cancer treatment currently well controlled?
2. What first- and/or second-line treatments has Mike tried, and how effective have they been?
3. Does Mike have any contraindications to cannabis treatment or precautions to consider?
4. If you decide to recommend medical cannabis for Mike, what formulation/product is appropriate?
5. Does Mike require any special monitoring based on his medical or medication history?

9.5.6 Assessment

Mike is seriously ill with stage IV cancer. He is undergoing multiple lines of chemotherapy, with disease progression and bone metastasis. He has cachexia, weight loss, nausea, and cancer pain but declines opioid pain medications. His goals are to be able to tolerate cancer treatment as long as he can and to reduce his pain and nausea to feel more comfortable, such as being able to take a few bites of his favorite foods and sleep in bed with his wife rather than sit up in a recliner chair due to pain and nausea. He says, "Doc, I'll take just one good day…one day without this pain."

Mike is a good candidate for medical cannabis treatment. He has stage IV cancer that is progressing despite cancer treatments, along with nausea, vomiting, weight loss, and cancer pain. His goals are clear, and there is evidence to support a trial of medical cannabis for his conditions, including some randomized controlled trials [8–11].

9.5.7   Recommendation

Given Mike's severe symptoms and prior cannabis experience, he is interested in a more rapid approach to relief. Since he has caregiver support and does not drive, you discuss starting a balanced formula with 2.5 mg CBD and 2.5 mg THC per dose (type II, 1:1 ratio THC/CBD).

9.5.8   Treatment Course, Counseling, and Monitoring

- The local dispensary has dissolvable troches in several flavors, starting at 2.5 mg CBD/2.5 mg THC per troche. Mike selects a cherry-flavored box and starts with one troche twice daily.
- At the 1-week follow-up visit, Mike reports that he has stopped vomiting, and his nausea is about half as severe. His pain has minimally improved. He starts his night in bed but still gets up after about 2 h due to pain. He denies impairment or sedation.
- Over the next week, he increases to a 5 mg CBD/5 mg THC troche twice daily. When he returns 2 weeks later, you see him smile for the first time. He has been able to take a bite of his wife's chocolate chip cookies once again, and it was "heaven." His pain has improved to his satisfaction during the day, but he is still restless and uncomfortable at night.
- Since he is tolerating the titration well, with good response and no adverse effects, you and Mike decide together to increase

his nighttime dose to two troches (10 mg CBD/10 mg THC total). He will keep the daytime dose the same at one troche.

- Two weeks later, Mike can now sleep 4 h in bed with his wife. He has been sipping milkshakes and taking a few bites of scrambled eggs and toast. His cancer treatment continues, and he is not pain-free, but he reports having "more energy for the fight" and is looking forward to more good days.

9.6   Case No. 6: Palliative and End-of-Life Care

9.6.1   Background/Chief Complaint

Josephine is an 81-year-old female who lives in a small private-assisted living facility. She is debilitated and bed-bound following a large stroke 3 years ago. Josephine's daughter recently heard a webinar about medical cannabis in the elderly and is wondering if it might help her mother be more comfortable and in less pain.

9.6.2   History of Present Illness

The stroke left Josephine with right-sided hemiparesis, expressive aphasia, and impaired swallowing. She hasn't been able to walk, sit up, or eat solid food since her stroke, and as a result, she has lost 60 pounds from her baseline weight of 155 pounds. Her physical condition has progressively deteriorated due to immobility and malnutrition, and she is now frail and cachectic, with painful contractures of her right arm and both legs. She also has skin breakdown and decubitus wounds on her sacrum and heels. She can be restless and agitated at night. When Josephine is awake, she cries out and grimaces in pain, especially during bathing and wound care. Sometimes, she swings her left arm at caregivers or pushes them away. Josephine can't feed herself but will eat a container of yogurt, pudding, or mashed potatoes when caregivers feed her. Most of her chronic medications have been stopped due to her swallowing issues and frailty, and she is only able to take small amounts of liquid medications.

Josephine's daughter recently met with a hospice company and is considering hospice care. Josephine's daughter says, "I know she is nearing the end; I just don't want her to suffer or be in pain."

9.6.3   Medical, Surgical, and Social History

Josephine's history includes hypertension, stroke, hypothyroidism, osteoporosis, and progressive dementia. Josephine's daughter shares that she is a very proud woman. Her husband and his brother both died while deployed in Vietnam, leaving her a widow with three children at 28 years old. She never remarried, and she went on to earn her nursing degree. She worked as a school nurse for 35 years before retiring. All of her children are grown, have gone to college, and are working with families of their own. She is beloved by her family, who are very close and supportive of her care and comfort.

9.6.4   Current Medications

Josephine had been taking metoprolol, aspirin, and levothyroxine for her chronic conditions; however, these have all been stopped in the past 2 months due to her frailty and swallowing issues.

9.6.5   Cannabis Use History and Preferences

To her daughter's knowledge, Josephine has never used cannabis.

Questions for the Clinician
Before reading further, pause to consider the following questions:

1. Are Josephine's symptoms currently well controlled?

2. What first-and/or second-line treatments has Josephine tried, and how effective have they been?
3. Does Josephine have any contraindications to cannabis treatment or precautions to consider?
4. If you decide to recommend medical cannabis for Josephine, what formulation/product is appropriate?
5. Does Josephine require any special monitoring based on her medical or medication history?

9.6.6   Assessment

End-of-life care is a unique specialty. Given the expected short prognosis of terminally ill patients, the focus of care at end-of-life shifts emphasizes patient preferences and comfort-centered interventions rather than curative treatments. Patients, caregivers, and providers alike all tend to be more open-minded and willing to explore complementary and alternative treatments that could improve comfort for individual patients. While evidence-based care remains the gold standard, additional modalities with limited evidence are often included in end-of-life care plans after risk/benefit discussions and identifying the goals of care.

Josephine may benefit from a trial of medical cannabis for her pain and restlessness. Positive treatment effects have been reported across multiple symptoms, including pain, nausea and vomiting, appetite, sleep, and agitation in dementia [12]. The usual challenges with interpretation remain relevant, with the majority of studies found to have a high risk of bias or low-quality evidence. The decision for a trial of medical cannabis in the palliative care setting should be a shared decision between the patient, caregivers, and clinician. As patients near the end of life, there is more openness to incorporating nontraditional treatments despite the lack of substantive evidence.

9.6.7   Recommendation

Josephine is unable to participate in a complex discussion about her care, and her daughter is her legal healthcare decision-maker. CBD (without THC) is an ideal starting point for Josephine. Its anti-inflammatory and anti-anxiety properties correlate well with Josephine's symptoms despite the lack of specific evidence. Another option that may help Josephine's pain and contractures without risk of impairment would be a topical cannabis formulation. Topical formulas absorb locally and there is some evidence that they reduce local pain [13]. THC should be avoided for Josephine due to her aphasia and agitation, with limited ability to monitor or screen for impairment or possible worsening of these symptoms.

9.6.8   Treatment Course, Counseling, and Monitoring

- Josephine's daughter purchased a flavorless CBD tincture from the dispensary, and she started administering 2.5 mg in her mother's yogurt or pudding twice daily.
- Josephine's daughter will try massaging her mother's arms and legs using a THC/CBD cream once daily.
- At the 1-and 2-week follow-ups, Josephine appears more relaxed without facial grimacing or moaning in pain. She still cries out during wound care, but in between those events, she is resting more comfortably. She really appears to enjoy the daily massages from her daughter and has even smiled during their time together. While it is hard to tell if the cannabis cream is effective, the loving touch and massages from her daughter have visibly improved Josephine's daily comfort.
- Josephine enters hospice care 4 weeks later and remains mostly comfortable as she becomes weaker and stops eating. Her needs for morphine, lorazepam, and other traditional comfort medications were limited to her final days of life, and her daughter was grateful for the improved time they had together.

References

1. Bergamaschi MM, Queiroz RH, Chagas MH, de Oliveira DC, De Martinis BS, Kapczinski F, Quevedo J, Roesler R, Schröder N, Nardi AE, Martín-Santos R, Hallak JE, Zuardi AW, Crippa JA. Cannabidiol reduces the anxiety induced by simulated public speaking in treatment-naïve social phobia patients. Neuropsychopharmacology. 2011;36:1216.
2. Velzeboer R, Malas A, Boerkoel P, Cullen K, Hawkins M, Roesler J, Lai WW. Cannabis dosing and administration for sleep: a systematic review. Sleep. 2022;45(11):zsac218. https://doi.org/10.1093/sleep/zsac218. Erratum in: Sleep. 2023 Mar 9;46(3):zsad008. doi: 10.1093/sleep/zsad008.
3. Baumeister SE, Baurecht H, Nolde M, Alayash Z, Gläser S, Johansson M, Amos CI, International Lung Cancer Consortium, Johnson EC, Hung RJ. Cannabis use, pulmonary function, and lung cancer susceptibility: a Mendelian randomization study. J Thorac Oncol. 2021;16(7):1127–35. https://doi.org/10.1016/j.jtho.2021.03.025. Epub 2021 Apr 20.
4. Karimian Azari E, Kerrigan A, O'Connor A. Naturally occurring cannabinoids and their role in modulation of cardiovascular health. J Diet Suppl. 2020;17(5):625–50. https://doi.org/10.1080/19390211.2020.1790708. Epub 2020 Jul 17.
5. Petzke F, Tölle T, Fitzcharles MA, Häuser W. Cannabis-based medicines and medical cannabis for chronic neuropathic pain. CNS Drugs. 2022;36(1):31–44. https://doi.org/10.1007/s40263-021-00879-w. Epub 2021 Nov 21. PMID: 34802112; PMCID: PMC8732831.
6. Dubois C, Danielson EC, Beestrum M, Eurich DT. Medical cannabis and its efficacy/effectiveness on the management of osteoarthritis pain and function. Curr Med Res Opin. 2024;40(7):1195–202. https://doi.org/10.1080/03007995.2024.2363945. Epub 2024 Jun 10.
7. McDonagh MS, Morasco BJ, Wagner J, Ahmed AY, Fu R, Kansagara D, Chou R. Cannabis-based products for chronic pain: a systematic review. Ann Intern Med. 2022;175(8):1143–53. https://doi.org/10.7326/M21-4520. Epub 2022 Jun 7.
8. Johnson JR, Burnell-Nugent M, Lossignol D, Ganae-Motan ED, Potts R, Fallon MT. Multicenter, double-blind, randomized, placebo-controlled, parallel-group study of the efficacy, safety, and tolerability of THC:CBD extract and THC extract in patients with intractable cancer-related pain. J Pain Symptom Manag. 2010;39(2):167–79. https://doi.org/10.1016/j.jpainsymman.2009.06.008. Epub 2009 Nov 5.
9. Zylla DM, Eklund J, Gilmore G, Gavenda A, Guggisberg J, VazquezBenitez G, Pawloski PA, Arneson T, Richter S, Birnbaum AK, Dahmer S, Tracy M, Dudek A. A randomized trial of medical cannabis in patients with stage IV cancers to assess feasibility, dose requirements, impact on pain and opioid use, safety, and overall patient satisfaction.

Support Care Cancer. 2021;29(12):7471–8. https://doi.org/10.1007/s00520-021-06301-x. Epub 2021 Jun 4.

10. Grimison P, Mersiades A, Kirby A, Lintzeris N, Morton R, Haber P, Olver I, Walsh A, McGregor I, Cheung Y, Tognela A, Hahn C, Briscoe K, Aghmesheh M, Fox P, Abdi E, Clarke S, Della-Fiorentina S, Shannon J, Gedye C, Begbie S, Simes J, Stockler M. Oral THC:CBD cannabis extract for refractory chemotherapy-induced nausea and vomiting: a randomised, placebo-controlled, phase II crossover trial. Ann Oncol. 2020;31(11):1553–60. https://doi.org/10.1016/j.annonc.2020.07.020. Epub 2020 Aug 13.

11. Chow R, Valdez C, Chow N, Zhang D, Im J, Sodhi E, Lock M. Oral cannabinoid for the prophylaxis of chemotherapy-induced nausea and vomiting-a systematic review and meta-analysis. Support Care Cancer. 2020;28(5):2095–103. https://doi.org/10.1007/s00520-019-05280-4. Epub 2020 Jan 8

12. Doppen M, Kung S, Maijers I, John M, Dunphy H, Townsley H, Eathorne A, Semprini A, Braithwaite I. Cannabis in palliative care: a systematic review of current evidence. J Pain Symptom Manag. 2022;64(5):e260–84. https://doi.org/10.1016/j.jpainsymman.2022.06.002. Epub 2022 Jun 12.

13. Grossman S, Tan H, Gadiwalla Y. Cannabis and orofacial pain: a systematic review. Br J Oral Maxillofac Surg. 2022;60(5):e677–90. https://doi.org/10.1016/j.bjoms.2021.06.005. Epub 2021 Jun 23.

Index

© The Editor(s) (if applicable) and The Author(s), under exclusive   143
license to Springer Nature Switzerland AG 2025
L. Sera, C. Hempel-Sanderoff, *Cannabis Science and Therapeutics*,
https://doi.org/10.1007/978-3-031-80352-9